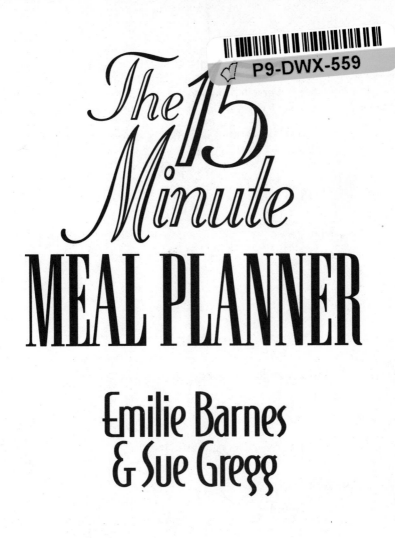

The 15 Minute
MEAL PLANNER

Emilie Barnes
& Sue Gregg

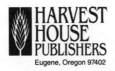

HARVEST
HOUSE
PUBLISHERS
Eugene, Oregon 97402

THE 15-MINUTE MEAL PLANNER

Copyright © 1994 by Harvest House Publishers
Eugene, Oregon 97402

Library of Congress Cataloging-in-Publication Data

Barnes, Emilie.
    The 15-minute meal planner / Emilie Barnes, Sue Gregg.
        p.   cm.
    ISBN 1-56507-234-0
    1. Cookery (Natural foods).   2. Nutrition.   3. Natural foods.
I. Gregg, Sue.   II. Title.   III. Title: Fifteen-minute meal planner.
TX741.B367   1994
641.5'63—dc20   94-30119
                                                                    CIP

Printed in the United States of America.

94 95 96 97 98 99 00 01 — 10 9 8 7 6 5 4 3 2 1

*To our husbands, Bob Barnes and Rich Gregg,
who have eaten everything in this book
and whose patience, support, and encouragement
have made this book possible,
and to the families who have found and will find
a new Eating Better Lifestyle.*

Introduction

Where is the busy woman who has enough time for her husband, children, work, fitness club, church, volunteer activities, rest, a good book, let alone her shopping and cooking? As more and more women have come to join the out-of-home work force, they have come to rely on prepackaged foods, frozen meals, dial-and-deliver meals, fast-food outlets, and restaurants for their family meals.

Today, however, thoughtful women are recognizing that convenience comes at a price. Convenience foods not only cost more; they also fill and fatten while failing to fulfill real nutrient needs. Health-conscious women now want to know how they can obtain nutritional quality along with convenience.

The 15-Minute Meal Planner was written to enable you to evaluate the vast array of food choices before you, to provide nutritional tips for making wise choices, and to put a realistic plan into action. The short chapters are designed to be read in 15 minutes or less. Take a chapter a day. Try one recipe at a time. And let those whom you serve reap the benefits of better health!

Contents

Meal Plans

Chart Index

Recipe List— by Category

(for index, see page 382)

9

PART 1

♥

How Did It All Begin?

♥

1

Emilie's Story

———— ❤ ————

$\mathcal{A}$s busy women we plan (or do not plan), shop, pre-pare, and cook over 750 meals per year. That is a major part of our lives. As I've been teaching More Hours in My Day seminars, one of the most frequently asked questions is "Where can I get ideas on balanced, nutritious meal planning, especially for my dinner meals?" We get into a rut with meals and need new, fresh ideas.

Fast-food restaurants are now preparing meals for us. For example, one major fast-food restaurant sells a triple cheeseburger with over 1,200 calories. Being overweight is a major problem for many people. Fad diets and diet books are bestsellers, and new fad diets pop up daily in magazines, newspapers, and books. How can we balance our health, weight, and the dilemma of the busy woman's meal planning? The answer is on the way!

First, though, let me tell you how it all began.

A Friday morning Bible study started when our son's best friend, Todd Miller, a 16-year-old professional moto-cross racer, was killed at the national championship race in Anaheim, California. Bob and Elaine's only child, gone. Tragedy and grief filled our neighborhood. Several of the neighborhood women suggested we start a support group Bible study in my home to help Elaine through the loss of

Todd. Up to 50 women attended with as many as 28 children in the nursery. God truly blessed as our lives were changed.

I'll never forget the first Friday morning that Sue Gregg came. A friend brought her. Two weeks earlier, Sue's three-year-old son, Stephen, was killed in the Greggs' front yard by a drunken teenage driver. Sue shared her story that day. We were blessed by Sue's testimony of comfort and peace despite the loss of her son.

Not long after coming to the Bible study, Sue attended one of my seminars. When I shared a short segment on proper foods and eating nature's way, I demonstrated the difference in size between a loaf of white bread and a loaf of whole-wheat bread by squeezing each from end to end. Sue's eyes lit up. A simple demonstration triggered her interest. God began a new work in her that day.

Now, let me go even further back.

My father, Otto Klein, was born and orphaned at a very early age in Vienna, Austria. At that time many European countries would place the orphans in areas where they could learn a vocation. My father had the wonderful opportunity of being placed in the kitchen in the Palace of Vienna where he worked side by side with some of the most famous chefs in the world. When he came as a young man to America, he came as a very fine Viennese chef. As the supervising chef, he opened many fine hotels and restaurants in the United States. In later years he worked for the movie studios and cooked for national and international celebrities.

My father cooked only with real butter, olive oil, and the very best natural ingredients. He always used brown rice and fresh vegetables. He considered catsup and canned or frozen foods a disgrace. He would receive compliments and standing ovations for his cooking. His secret was using high-grade natural ingredients with creative flair and quality perfection.

During my early years I ate nothing but the best of foods—not necessarily rich, but whole and natural. We had little as far as material possessions, but we did eat well. Daddy always said, "We are what we eat." The only recipes I have remembered from childhood are those I watched him cook as I sat on the drain board in our tiny kitchen with its icebox and small gas stove.

When my father died, I was 11 years old. My mother then became a single working parent of two children. With borrowed money she opened up a small dress shop. I grew up behind my mother's shop in three tiny rooms.

After marrying my teenage sweetheart, Bob Barnes, I became a mother of five children under five years of age. I was only 21. Three of the children were my brother's. His wife had walked out the door abandoning them all, and he could not take care of them. The years that followed gave me experience in preparing thousands of meals. We developed a natural-foods lifestyle. With balanced nutrition our family was healthy, and yet the food was always tasty. We are not health nuts. We do eat chocolate chip cookies and waffles with maple syrup occasionally. We even enjoy chips and dip.

God has given me a heart's desire to teach women to be makers of their homes (Titus 2:4,5). Sue and I will share with you our secrets of tasty, nutritious, low-cost meals that you can prepare as busy women in a fast-food world. You'll have more time, energy, and health to do the things you've always wanted to do. You will be blessed as you survive in a busy world with more hours in *your* day. We will answer questions on eating out: where to go and what to order. We have prepared three dinner meal plans with recipe selections to get you started with the *Eating Better Lifestyle:* a 25-Day Unlimited Meal Plan, a 19-Day No-Meat Plan, and a 19-Day No-Dairy, No-Egg Plan. Our recipes have passed the taste test of family and friends, receiving many compliments, too. They will add to your joy of cooking.

2

Sue's Story

———— ♥ ————

I've always been interested in food preparation. My first
serious venture was in high school home economics
when I selected two weeks of planning and preparing family dinners as my special project. Not long after this, I was
invited to plan and supervise the food service at a church
retreat. Pursuing this interest, I enrolled in a university
home economics program. In my freshman year I became a
Christian through a dorm Bible study. It took me many
years to understand, however, that what I learned through
academic training too often ignored the values God had
created in food.

Armed with a teaching credential, I taught two years of
junior high and high school home economics. Meal planning centered on the Basic Four food groups. Appetite
interest was enhanced by variety in color, tastes, textures,
and temperatures. It was all based upon the use of white
flour, white sugar, hydrogenated fats, meat as the main
dish, and prepackaged and canned foods. In addition to
teaching and feeding my growing family, I was asked to
manage the food service for many camps and retreats. That
included seven beautiful summers at Campus by the Sea on
Catalina Island where I received invaluable experience

serving the American Diet to varying tastes of all ages in a facility without electricity or adequate refrigeration.

My awareness of the nutritional value of food began when I was pregnant with our fourth child. Inspired by Adele Davis's *Let's Have Healthy Children*, I managed to break the bottle barrier and nurse little Stephen for nine months. However, when he was a year old, he began to contract a series of sniffles and colds that sent us to the doctor. There I was supplied with antibiotics which I faithfully administered for ten full prescribed days on each occurrence. The runny nose didn't stop. I began to question, "Didn't God create Stephen's body with an immune system that could fight off infection and disease?" I decided to stop running to the doctor for every little sniffle. Eventually my son's immune system took care of the problem. That gave me more incentive to find ways to help my family prevent and fight illness as the first measure and make antibiotics and drugs the second measure.

In my research I discovered that some great gaps exist in the world between those who have little to eat and those who have an abundance. The irony is that both are hungry. The hunger of the first group is for a satisfied stomach. The unknown hunger of the second group (including myself and everyone else eating the American Diet) is for the nutritional values that technology has removed from the whole-food sources. Reading Frances Moore Lappe's *Diet for a Small Planet*, I determined to do something about the world hunger problem. I read about how much grain it took to feed cattle so that affluent societies could enjoy a meat-centered diet. I tried some of the alternative meatless recipes on my family without success. My husband, Rich, was a meat-and-potatoes man, and even at age two our Stephen was a meat lover! The other children didn't get excited about tasteless bean-and-grain casseroles, either.

One day as I stood at my kitchen sink, I prayed, "Lord, is my interest in world hunger and nutrition wrong? Should I just forget about it?" In my mind a quiet, small voice prompted, "No, you are on the right track, but your timing is off, and your attitude is wrong. Trust Me, keep on researching and learning. Allow Me to change your attitude and give your husband and children receptivity to this new venture." I set aside my meatless meal experiments.

Soon a traumatic event changed the course of our lives. As our three-year-old Stephen was playing on the front lawn with his two older sisters, a drunken teenage driver proceeded slowly down our street and struck our utility trailer and car. The trailer slammed over the curb and hit Stephen in the head as the driver continued down the street. While my husband breathed air into Stephen's limp, bleeding form, all I could pray was, "Jesus, help!"

Indeed, God does minister to our loss and grief through His miraculous gift of grace, love, and comfort. After a graveside service, we shared a meal with close friends and family. One dear friend shared a passage of Scripture that was to become a cornerstone for our ministry. Isaiah 58:6-12 speaks of "spending yourselves on behalf of the hungry." Often during the 17 years that have passed, my husband and I have returned to study that passage to remind ourselves of God's purpose and direction as we research, publish, and teach about food.

Within a few days one caring Christian neighbor sent a note expressing her concern. Encouraged, I visited her and shared our experience of God's comfort in our sorrow. She invited me to share my story with her Friday morning Bible study group which met at Emilie Barnes's home.

Several months later, Emilie Barnes and Florence Littauer held a seminar on how to be a godly woman in the home. Emilie included a ten-minute talk about nutrition. When she mashed a loaf of fluffy white bread into a mangled mass, I was impressed. She didn't just stop with the squeeze. Pricking the ballooning plastic bread bag, she exploded it. It was evident that the number-one ingredient in that loaf of bread was air, and what was left was at best calories with only a fraction of the original nutrients. Emilie dramatized what I was already beginning to discover about food. In fact, I had already purchased a bread kneader and flour mill and was preparing whole-wheat breads, cinnamon rolls, and pizza for my family. My children and husband loved them! That was God's way of bringing change to my family. That day my dream to minister to women in the area of food and nutrition was born.

I began to read all of the books and articles on food preparation and nutrition that I could find. Rich, too, became interested. In fact, he took some tests and found out that he was actually a borderline diabetic! This unexpected revelation launched us into an even more serious investigation of how to change family food patterns. It seemed incredible that I hadn't learned these things during five years of home economics courses.

I began to read labels. My daughter Karen and I scoured the cupboards for all the questionable packaged foods, put them in a corner cupboard, and tied a string around the handles. We put ourselves to the test. If we could survive two weeks without these foods, perhaps we could do so for life. We did and we still do.

I learned how to prepare foods more complete in nutritional value. I learned about the values of fresh fruits and vegetables over canned, and how to fix a dinner without meat. Inevitably other people began to ask about the changes my family was making in food choices. As I began to share my whole-grain breads, friends asked for the recipes. Informal kitchen sessions grew into demonstration classes. A few handout recipes expanded into two editions of *Natural Foods for All Occasions*, a recipe newsletter, the **Eating Better Cookbooks**, and a cooking demonstration video, *Eating Better with Sue*.

Our family experienced positive results. My husband's prediabetic condition was quickly corrected. He lost excess weight and gained back his livable and loving disposition. His energy began to return. Dreams and goals supplanted depression. My son's frequent headaches and earaches diminished. Frequent visits to the doctor virtually ceased for all of us.

We realize that every aspect of our lives affects health and that nutritional change is not a guarantee of optimum health. Whatever the results, <u>our desire is to reflect God's life-giving purpose for food in</u> what we do with it. We have no intention of reverting back to the American Diet. We are committed because we believe that God has designed a life-giving nutritional plan for our benefit.

In addition to nutritional research, Rich and I began to investigate what the Bible had to say about food. With a concordance we checked out every reference we could find in the Bible about food or applicable to food. We found an incredible wealth of biblical principles, although not many recipes or menus. God knew what He was doing when He designed bodies and then created food for them. Our appreciation of Him as Creator and Provider expanded.

<u>Every member of my family</u> has not only benefited from the change but has also <u>learned</u> how to prepare wholesome <u>foods.</u> My son, Dan, has specialized in bread baking and served as a part-time cook in a college whole-foods cafeteria. Karen, my older daughter, loves international cookery, is an excellent soup maker, and arranges beautiful fresh salads. Sharon, the youngest, is a real organizer in putting a whole meal together and serving it attractively, plus she bakes whole-grain cookies and healthy desserts. Now married, she carries on the tradition of <u>healthy meal planning</u> in her own home using my menu planning system and cookbooks, plus her own creative style. And she was our picky eater! Her husband, Duane, is truly blessed. Her dream is to have a Bed-and-Breakfast. Our son, Dan, and his wife, Valerie, have given us our first grandson, Yosef—a bundle of life and energy. At 17 months he does not walk—he runs! As Dan said during Valerie's pregnancy, "Our baby has been getting a healthy diet with lots of whole-grain bread and no junk food, except a cookie or two that Valerie ate." <u>The skills of food choice and preparation,</u>

unfortunately, have been lost to most of the current generation. That is why my husband and I have committed ourselves to teaching others how to make the transition to eating better.

I appreciate the ideas that Emilie's smashed loaf of bread sparked. This demonstration helped me believe that it was possible to lead people from imitations to real God-given, life-producing food. With that same faith I believe that we can take charge of our lives—the way we eat, work, play, rest, minister to others, and worship.

3

Setting the Scene

———— ♥ ————

In the beginning God created the heavens and the earth. . . . God saw all that he had made, and it was very good.

Genesis 1:1,31

———— ♥ ————

This book has been written for one simple reason: We can eat better. Our families can eat better, too. Why? Because the typical twentieth-century American diet no longer adequately contains the nutritional value that God originally created in food. Current medical and scientific research has amply demonstrated that we are reaping the consequences in a host of daily health problems, degenerative diseases, and untimely deaths.

This should come as no surprise. Whenever mankind alters or ignores God's resources for life and health, tragic consequences follow. What a dishonor to Him who intended food to do good and not evil to mankind! He intended that the food He made for us would, instead, reap the benefits of health and well-being. It is that simple.

24

Yet we cannot promise you sensational health transformations. We cannot promise that you will lose 50 pounds, never get colds again, or never get cancer, heart disease, or diabetes. We cannot promise you that your energy will automatically soar. These and many other health benefits can and will happen to many people. Better nutrition will help each one of us where better nutrition is what our health needs. But since our health depends upon a whole complex of genetic, environmental, relational, and habitual lifestyle conditions, the benefits of eating better will vary widely. Nevertheless, nutrition does make a difference in the quality of our lives. And since God created food to be the vehicle of that nutrition, we honor Him when we pay attention to and utilize food's nutritional quality. We dishonor Him when we ignore good nutrition.

We believe that you will find this book unique in several ways. We do not expect our readers to treat the nutritional importance of food in an isolated or rigid way. Food means more than nutrition. It means family fellowship and celebration. It means security and comfort. It means cultural identity. It means giving, receiving, and sharing love. It is unrealistic to strive for better eating for nutrition's sake if these values that we place upon food are ignored, overlooked, or sacrificed. Therefore, we have approached this subject of eating better in the broader context of the role that food plays in our lives.

For example, the American dietary pattern is part of our cultural inheritance and is thus not easily abandoned for a strange diet, no matter how nutritious it may be. Hamburgers, spaghetti, pizza, and meat and potatoes are still in, but we can improve the nutritional quality through better choices of ingredients.

Many books attempt to achieve the ultimate in nutritional purity so that the many dos and don'ts lead to restriction rather than freedom. This leads to discouragement and failure. We want to introduce you to a wide range of choices you can enjoy with food of greater nutritional quality. We admit that we don't know everything there is to know about nutrition. Nobody does. There is controversy on many points. Therefore, we encourage you to make basic changes that have been well-established by scientific research. Then consider the range of choices we offer about the controversial issues. We will present you with these options rather than merely give you our own views as if they were the last word on the subject.

We do not pretend that the lifestyle change to eating better is simple. It is not. If you are to make lasting and permanent changes, you will need to make choices that will work well within the framework of your own circumstances. It will require commitment and perseverance to overcome obstacles. Some of these barriers are fears that can be allayed through better understanding. These are 1) How is it all going to taste? Will my family like it? 2) How much time is required to focus on eating better? 3) How will it affect my food budget? and 4) Where can the food resources be purchased? Other concerns are how to get started, how to help your family change, and how to choose better food when eating out.

Most women want practical help. This translates into where to buy the food, what to buy, and what recipes and menus to use. All the nutritional information in the world will not help if you do not have these resources. In Part 7 you will find dinner meal plans, the recipes and menus to prepare them, and the help you need to buy the ingredients. If you are ready to start, don't wait to read all the nutrition and biblical background sections. Read Parts 2 and 3, Our Cultural Food Heritage and Coping with Change, for perspective and encouragement. Then you can treat Parts 4 and 5 (the background sections) as a small encyclopedia, if you wish. Look up the answers to your questions as they arise while you are choosing and preparing the recipes and menus. The *"Eating Better with Sue"* video cooking course also incorporates readings and recipes from this book with the lessons (see p. 383).

God has set before us both life and death, and He calls us to choose life. Therefore, He will assist you in every way that you need to overcome obstacles to eating better. Every step you take will count for life. Look at your progress and be thankful for that, rather than focusing on what still hasn't been done. God loves you infinitely and is willing to honor your commitment. Get organized and start moving. Do it with prayer. Your health and the health of your family is important to God. He desires to use you in our needy world to bring glory and honor to His name. To do that you need all the health and strength and vigor you can acquire.

That brings us to our final perspective in this book. It is biblically based. The health-food movement has been primarily associated with the New Age Movement, bringing in Eastern, Hinduistic philosophies. We will say more about this in later chapters. Here we want to note that when we see nutrition books that are associated with this philosophy of life on the shelves of Christian bookstores, we believe a confrontive biblical approach is needed.

There is much confusion in many believers' minds about the relationship of body and spirit. Few people recognize that the problem of eating better is an issue of spiritual warfare. Here are some reasons why we know this to be true. Physical food was God's first gift to mankind. He involved food's use in His test of man's obedience. Satan used food as an enticement for man's rebellion against Him. The Israelites' rebellion against God in the wilderness concerned food. Jesus' first temptation by the devil in the wilderness was a food temptation. The first contention that arose in the early church was over a matter of food distribution. The expression of the most important spiritual truth of all time—that Jesus Christ died on the cross for sins—is represented by the food symbols of bread and wine, established by Jesus Christ Himself.

Satan is a thief who steals, kills, and destroys. If he can do it through nutritionally poor food, which he is doing on a grand scale, he will. If he can do it by associating anti-Christian philosophies with good food, he will do that, too. And, I might add, he is having a heyday playing his

role on the other side of the nutritional "fence" by suggesting all manner of restrictions through a host of nutrition
enthusiasts and technocrats who focus on the "don't eats":
Don't eat salt, don't eat fat, don't eat meat, don't drink
milk . . . don't, don't, don't. The list grows, making healthful eating unappetizing and too difficult—just what Satan
wants! We need to prayerfully ask God for discernment.

The following chapters introduce you to a broad variety
of nutritional and practical food issues, many of which we
have mentioned in this chapter. Where we have found
other books to be good resources on a particular topic, we
have named those at appropriate places. These references
have then been listed together on a Recommended Reading
list on pp. 379-81. We encourage you to get involved right
away in the action in Part 6 with recipes and menus as you
read this book.

4

What Are the Benefits?

---------- ♥ ----------

He himself gives all men life and breath and everything else. . . . For in him we live and move and have our being.

Acts 17:25,28

---------- ♥ ----------

*T*he measure of health one has is dependent upon a healthy system of digestion and elimination. All the other processes of the body are strengthened by it—the immune, circulatory, and lymphatic systems, for example. We fail to appreciate these benefits fully because we cannot see them happening. But we can appreciate the results in our daily lives. Eating a healthy balance of life-giving food will contribute to benefits that we all desire:

- ♥ Better weight control
- ♥ More youthful appearance—healthier skin, hair, eyes
- ♥ More energy
- ♥ Greater mental alertness

- ♥ More stable emotions
- ♥ Freedom from common digestive discomforts
- ♥ Increased resistance to illness
- ♥ Increased resistance to degenerative diseases
- ♥ Faster and more complete healing of injuries
- ♥ Slower aging—longer life

These benefits will also result in:

- ♥ Less money needed for medical bills
- ♥ Less time spent in bed, in doctors' offices, in hospitals
- ♥ More freedom to enjoy and love family and friends
- ♥ More freedom for ministry and service to God

PART 2

♥

Our Cultural Food Heritage

♥

5

Grandpa Ate Everything and Lived to 92!

———— ♥ ————

He makes grass grow for the cattle, and plants for man to cultivate—bringing forth food from the earth: wine that gladdens the heart of man, oil to make his face shine, and bread that sustains his heart.

Psalm 104:14,15

———— ♥ ————

Someone's hale-and-hearty grandpa always managed to have enjoyed eating what he liked on his journey to a ripe old age! If he could do it, why can't I? How did Grandpa manage? To answer that we must hearken back to Grandpa's childhood on the family farm.

Grandpa was a hardworking young man from the time he could collect the daily egg quota. No time for lying down on the job. The cows needed milking, the garden needed weeding, the crops needed harvesting. School and studies took up the evening hours. There were special occasions, though, for socializing, fun, and feasting. These were big events and included the usual broad spread of farm-fresh beef, pork, chicken, fresh vegetables, homemade gravy, fresh hot rolls with lots of churned butter, milk, and hot apple, cherry, and pumpkin pies with homemade ice cream. In fact, everyday meals were a simplified version of such feasts as these, calculated to satisfy the appetites of farmers who worked from dawn till dusk.

In Grandpa's day the air in the country was fresh, clear, and unpolluted. The water from the creek was pure. Pesticides and herbicides were unheard of. Farm-fresh produce was organic and uncontaminated. Seasonal produce brought ripe from vine and tree to the dining table was a way of life. The foods you didn't grow on your own, you often did not have to eat. Available meats and poultry were lean and free of antibiotics and growth stimulants. Fish came from unpolluted streams and rivers. Although meats, fish, and poultry were available, if Grandpa lived at the turn of the century, he was probably eating more of his protein in beans, grains, and vegetables.

There were lean times, too. The Depression years provided an especially prolonged time of frugal fare. Hearty eating was not always one long and unending feast from birth to the grave. Lean times may well have provided many digestive systems with a needed respite from more sumptuous seasons. The daily struggles against the caprice of the elements provided experiences that firmed up resolve and fortitude. Family values, social and moral standards, and the work ethic were all more clearly delineated, understood, and lived by. All of these living patterns contributed to Grandpa's hale-and-hearty condition.

Alas! Grandpa's world is no longer our world. In fact, not too many grandpas or favorite old uncles are living to a ripe old age anymore, at least not without the typical health traumas of cancers, heart attacks, diabetes, and Alzheimer's disease. What has happened? How has our world and food supply changed? What have we inherited?

6

Whatever Happened to the Basic Four?

———— ♥ ————

I brought you into a fertile land to eat its fruit and rich produce. But you came and defiled my land and made my inheritance detestable.

Jeremiah 2:7

———— ♥ ————

*G*randpa was not too concerned with the nutrition in his food. He just ate and lived or ate and got sick, most often from something other than what was lacking in his food. His food may not have been perfect, but there were many other contributions to health in his life to compensate for what was lacking. Grandpa got what nutrients he could because much of what he needed still remained intact in his food. Although he certainly was consuming some white flour and white sugar in a variety of recipes, his generation was not yet reaping the full effect of food devitalization. Fresh and lean farm products also helped to make up for this lack. Practically everything he ate was freshly prepared in the home kitchen. Almost all of the young women in his day learned how to cook from basic foods.

The first vitamin, vitamin B_2, was not discovered until 1886 by Casimir Funk. A full quarter of our twentieth century was gone before Albert Szent-Gyorgyi discovered vitamin C. Gyorgyi expressed appropriate appreciation. "Vitamins . . . will help us to reduce human suffering to an extent which the most fantastic mind would fail to imagine."[1] Of course, the Creator imagined it from the beginning and knew all along what He had put into food for our benefit. The discoveries of nutritional research have mushroomed since Gyorgyi's discovery.

As new information about food was learned, new tools for educating the American population were developed. The Basic Seven food groups were classified as a practical guideline to planning nutritious meals. Later, the Basic Seven was simplified to the Basic Four food groups. Specific size and number of servings were designated for each food group. The plan was easy to follow because it focused on groups of actual foods that could be harvested, stored, prepared, and tasted, rather than on nutrients hidden in the foods.

The Basic Four plan was ideal in a rural economy. The food groups very simply reflected farm fare—meats, fish, poultry, eggs, beans; dairy products; fruits and vegetables; and breads and cereals.

Another food revolution was about to occur. The advent of modern food technology ushered in supermarket shelves full of new food products of which white flour and white sugar of the previous century were only a forerunner. Most of these new products were and are different versions of the same theme—refined foods such as white flour and white sugar, stripped of major portions of fiber and nutrients, and dressed up with a wide variety of chemicals that never were part of the original food. Twinkies and Fruit Loops joined the home-baked white breads and pie crusts. Public consumption of these new products began to escalate. In addition, cattlemen were beginning to develop new ways to produce juicier and more tender meats. As the population was migrating to the cities, there was an increased need for fruits and vegetables preserved for those who didn't grow their own. An increasing variety of fruits and vegetables commercially canned in sugar syrups or with salt entered the market.

Unfortunately, most of these new food products fit neatly into the Basic Four food groups. Someone could eat the proper daily allotment of the Basic Four by having juicy beef filled with antibiotics and excessive fat, canned fruits in sugar syrup, salty canned vegetables, processed American cheese, chocolate ice cream, white toast, Fruit Loops, and Twinkies. Thousands upon thousands of food products developed since World War II made it not only possible, but a reality in most American households for people to get plenty to eat while eating relatively few basic whole foods.

It was apparent that a different food plan was needed to give adequate guidance for selecting nutritious foods and menus. The chart below illustrates the typical American diet. The *Eating Better Lifestyle* chart illustrates our recommended changes. The contrast between the typical American diet and the *Eating Better Lifestyle* is summarized in the charts on pp. 38-40. The meal plans, recipes, and menu suggestions in Part 7 reflect the guidelines of the *Eating Better Lifestyle*.

In 1990, the USDA answered the need for a different food plan by replacing the Basic Four with the Food Guide Pyramid (p. 41).

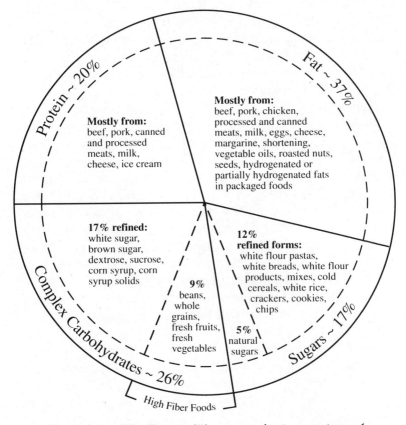

Protein ~ 20%

Mostly from:
beef, pork, canned
and processed
meats, milk,
cheese, ice cream

Fat ~ 37%

Mostly from:
beef, pork, chicken,
processed and canned
meats, milk, eggs, cheese,
margarine, shortening,
vegetable oils, roasted nuts,
seeds, hydrogenated or
partially hydrogenated fats
in packaged foods

Complex Carbohydrates ~ 26%

17% refined:
white sugar,
brown sugar,
dextrose, sucrose,
corn syrup, corn
syrup solids

9%
beans,
whole
grains,
fresh fruits,
fresh
vegetables

12%
refined forms:
white flour pastas,
white breads, white flour
products, mixes, cold
cereals, white rice,
crackers, cookies,
chips

5%
natural
sugars

Sugars ~ 17%

High Fiber Foods

The American Diet. Percents (%) are approximate percentages of calories.

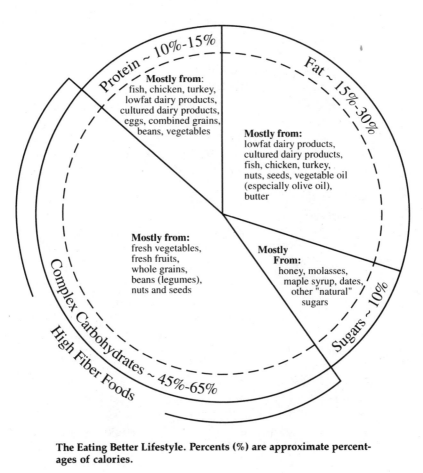

Protein ~ 10%-15%

Mostly from: fish, chicken, turkey, lowfat dairy products, cultured dairy products, eggs, combined grains, beans, vegetables

Fat ~ 15%-30%

Mostly from: lowfat dairy products, cultured dairy products, fish, chicken, turkey, nuts, seeds, vegetable oil (especially olive oil), butter

Mostly from: fresh vegetables, fresh fruits, whole grains, beans (legumes), nuts and seeds

Mostly From: honey, molasses, maple syrup, dates, other "natural" sugars

Sugars ~ 10%

Complex Carbohydrates ~ 45%-65%

High Fiber Foods

The Eating Better Lifestyle. Percents (%) are approximate percentages of calories.

TAKING A LOOK AT THE DIFFERENCE

THE TYPICAL AMERICAN DIET

- ♥ High in meat and dairy foods
- ♥ High in refined carbohydrates
- ♥ Low in unrefined carbohydrates
- ♥ 4000–6000 mg. sodium/day
- ♥ HIGH FAT—LOW FIBER

Deficient (or devitalized): Refined carbohydrates are deficient in original fiber, vitamins, minerals, and unknown nutritional properties. Refined oils have lost many nutrients.

Unbalanced: Excessive refined sugars and starches, fats, meat and dairy protein, and sodium (4000–6000 milligrams per day).

Adulterated: A large portion of these foods contains many added chemicals suspect to human health—pesticide residues, preservatives, artificial colorings, and flavorings.

Altered: Especially oils through processing, oxidation, cooking, hydrogenation.

EATING BETTER LIFESTYLE

- ♥ Low in meat and dairy foods
- ♥ Low in refined carbohydrates
- ♥ High in unrefined carbohydrates
- ♥ Less than 2400 mg. sodium/day
- ♥ LOW FAT—HIGH FIBER

The menus and recipes on pp. 309-74 aim toward developing the *Eating Better Lifestyle* pattern.

More complete nutrient supply: More whole (unrefined) complex carbohydrate foods and fats contain more original fiber, vitamins, minerals, and unknown nutritional properties.

Better balance: Less refined sugars and starches, fat, meat protein, and sodium (less than 2400 mg. per day).

Less adulterated: A large portion of these foods contains a significantly lower amount of chemicals suspect to human health.

Not altered: Oils in liquid form, less refined, utilizing oils appropriate for the purpose.

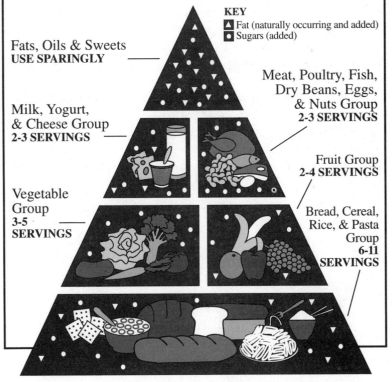

Food Guide Pyramid
A Guide to Daily Food Choices

Fats, Oils & Sweets
USE SPARINGLY

KEY
▲ Fat (naturally occurring and added)
● Sugars (added)

Meat, Poultry, Fish,
Dry Beans, Eggs,
& Nuts Group
2-3 SERVINGS

Milk, Yogurt,
& Cheese Group
2-3 SERVINGS

Fruit Group
2-4 SERVINGS

Vegetable
Group
**3-5
SERVINGS**

Bread, Cereal,
Rice, & Pasta
Group
**6-11
SERVINGS**

The Food Guide Pyramid: A guide to daily food choices (U.S. Department of Agriculture, U.S. Department of Health and Human Services).

The best asset of the Food Guide Pyramid is its visual impression—that grains, fruits, and vegetables should provide the bulk of the diet, supplemented with smaller amounts of meat and dairy products, and using small amounts of fats and sugars. Certainly this is an improvement over the Basic Four food groups.

Is the Food Guide Pyramid an adequate guide for meeting the goals of the *Eating Better Lifestyle*? Based on the suggested number of servings in each food group, carbohydrates (bread and cereal group plus fruit and vegetable groups) would provide about 55% of the diet. Protein (meat and dairy groups) would provide about 20%. The Pyramid approaches the need for increased carbohydrates, yet without specifying "whole" or "unrefined carbohydrates." According to our suggested *Eating Better* plan, the suggested amount of animal protein is still too high.

All charts that merely list foods and percentages, however, whether complete or incomplete, must be translated into daily menus and meal-plan combinations. In addition to those in Part 6, the *Eating Better Cookbooks* (see p. 383) offer 200 menus combined into ten meal plans that meet our *Eating Better Lifestyle* goals.

7

God's Cornucopia of Whole Foods

———— ♥ ————

Then God said, "I give you every seed-bearing plant on the face of the whole earth and every tree that has fruit with seed in it. They will be yours for food. . . . Everything that lives and moves will be food for you. Just as I gave you the green plants, I now give you everything."
Genesis 1:29; 9:3

———— ♥ ————

*W*hen Sue was developing a whole-foods quantity program for a college cafeteria, she requested some evaluations. One student responded, "Health food is not in the Bible." He included a series of Scriptures to prove the point! This evaluation reflected the idea that biblically there are no right foods to eat, especially not ones that you don't like!

We agree that there are many health-food products and recipes from health-food cookbooks that don't taste very good—at least not to the American palate. That, however, is an evaluation of the recipes used, not of the basic food ingredients used in the products. Most health-food products do use basic food ingredients that are closer to the way God made them than typical American food fare. In this sense, health food most certainly is in the Bible. But our understanding and, indeed, our appreciation for basic whole foods will be enhanced if we can separate them from the man-produced recipes and menus they are used in. Making the basic whole foods tasty in recipes and menus is a separate issue and the subject of the next chapter.

Let's look at God's cornucopia of whole foods generally available to most Americans, either seasonally or year-round. There are available in our culture approximately:

15 *Whole Grains*—amaranth, barley, brown rice, buckwheat, cornmeal, Kamut, oats, millet, quinoa, rye, sorghum, spelt, teff, triticale, wheat

17 *Legumes* (dry beans and peas)—azuki, black, black-eyed, carob, fava, garbanzo, great nothern, kidney, lentils, lima, mung, navy, peanuts, pinto, red, soy, split pea

18 *Nuts and Seeds*—alfalfa seeds, almonds, Brazil nuts, caraway seeds, cashews, chia seeds, coconut, filberts, flax seeds, macadamia nuts, pecans, pine nuts, pistachio nuts, poppy seeds, pumpkin seeds, sesame seeds, sunflower seeds, walnuts

60 *Fresh Vegetables*

33 *Fresh Fruits*

7 *Dairy Products*—butter, cream, cultured milks, eggs, hard cheeses, soft cheeses, sweet milk

4 *Meats and Poultry*—beef, chicken, lamb, turkey

20 *Fish*

20 *Herbs and Spices* (at least)

10 Tasty, Wholesome Sweeteners—barley malt syrup, date sugar, honey, maple sugar, maple syrup, molasses, rice syrup, sorghum syrup, stevia (an herbal sweetener), whole sugar cane (i.e. *Sucanat*)

This is just the variety of food commonly available in our own country! Imagine the many varieties in other cultures that we know little about. There are many different kinds of even one food—bananas, for example. Think for a moment, if you will, of the many ways in which these basic foods can be prepared and combined in recipes and menus. The exponential possibilities are staggering!

Is it not wonderful that God chose to give us such food variety to work with? He so easily could have provided us only with manna just as He did for the Israelites in the wilderness for 40 years. But it is evident that God loves variety and has lavishly displayed it in creation. It reflects the awesomeness of His glory and power. God's Word tells us that His "invisible qualities—his eternal power and divine nature—have been clearly seen, being understood from what has been made" (Romans 1:20). Imagine it! We are called upon to recognize God's eternal power and divine nature from the food He has created! How is that possible if the foods we eat are so devitalized* and adulterated* that they are significant contributors to such things as cancers, heart disease, diabetes, overweight, and a host of other unhappy ills? The chart on p. 46 illustrates this. On the contrary, foods are meant to give life because they originated out of the invisible qualities of our life-giving God. If we, His children, are to reflect the character of our heavenly Father, then we too must seek to utilize food in a life-giving way. He has provided us with a wealth of life-giving whole foods in order to do that.

---

* *Devitalized* means that many of the life-giving nutrients have been processed out of the food. *Adulterated* means that chemicals not originally in the food have been added for preservation, coloring, and flavoring.

Whole Wheat: A Lesson in Nutritional Loss

Nutrients Available in Whole-Wheat Flour	Nutrient Loss in All-Purpose White Flour[1]
Vitamins	
thiamine (B_1)*	77%
riboflavin (B_2)*	67%
niacin (B_3)*	81%
pyridoxine (B_6)	72%
choline (part of B-complex)	30%
folic acid (part of B-complex)	67%
pantothenic acid (part of B-complex)	50%
vitamin E	86%
Minerals	
chromium	40%
manganese	86%
selenium	16%
zinc	98%
iron*	75%
cobalt	89%
calcium	60%
sodium	78%
potassium	77%
magnesium	85%
phosphorus	91%
molybdenum	48%
copper	68%
Total average loss	70%

*These nutrients are added to "enriched" white flour in synthetic form, but are not restored in the original natural form. *Dietary Fiber:* 1 cup whole-wheat flour = 15.1 grams; 1 cup white flour = 2.9 grams (81% loss). *Nutrient value of wheat germ and bran is unknown.*

Approximately 50% of the American Diet is refined carbohydrate. Most of it is in the form of these
food items prepared from all-purpose white flour:

> noodles, spaghetti, macaroni, lasagna noodles,
> cake mixes, cookie mixes, pancake mixes, fro-
> zen waffles, breakfast cereals, sandwich breads,
> hot dog buns, hamburger buns, English muf-
> fins, flour tortillas, pita breads, bread mixes,
> prepackaged pasta mixes, pizza, crackers, cakes,
> cookies, doughnuts, croissants, sweet rolls,
> muffins, biscuit and roll mixes, dinner rolls

A good portion of refined carbohydrate also comes
from white rice and degerminated cornmeal, white rice
mixes, cornmeal mixes, corn tortillas, and corn chips devitalized in the same way as white flour.

8

The Recipe Box— Using God's Resources Imaginatively

———— ♥ ————

Let us make man in our image, in our likeness, and let them rule over the fish of the sea and the birds of the air, over the livestock, over all the earth, and over all the creatures that move along the ground.

Genesis 1:26

———— ♥ ————

*H*ave you ever wondered why there are many listings of foods in the Bible but few, if any, recipes and menus? Obviously the creation of recipes, menus, and cookbooks is our privileged domain. More cookbooks are published and sold than books in any other subject category. The endless variety of recipes from family to family, region to region, and culture to culture reflects how well we imitate the Creator!

Now we have the opportunity to fulfill the divine design by choosing the best of God's whole-food provisions and by handling those foods with care. The standard we've chosen for the recipes in this book comes from Deuteronomy 30:19,20: "Now choose life, so that you and your children may live. . . . For the LORD is your life, and he will give you many years in the land." It is our aim to constantly be alert to new food sources, new food preparation techniques, and food combinations in recipes and menus that maximize the life-giving benefits of God's wonderful provision.

At the same time we are aware that a brief encounter with "health foods" (foods that are "good" for you) has provided many with their first and decidedly last encounter. There are two reasons why. First, health-food advocates have often forgotten that taste buds have no brains. That means that appetites are whet by sensual responses, not by nutritional analyses. Secondly, health foods too often begin with the unfamiliar (e.g. macrobiotic or vegetarian) rather than with familiar foods.

Every cultural group has a distinct dietary pattern. While there is great diversity in the cultural backgrounds of Americans, there is an American pattern (witness the same menus served by restaurant chains from coast to coast and even overseas!) as opposed, say, to a Japanese or Mexican pattern. In the recipes and menus in this book we've chosen not to abandon all the American favorites, but to improve the quality of the familiar while introducing the new. The chart on page 50 illustrates what a difference just improving the ingredients of one familiar recipe—our *Minute Blender Bran Muffins* (p. 356) can make!

Taste and appetite are God-given, just as the indispensable nutrients in food are God-given. The challenge to us is to create a variety of recipes and menus that offer both.

Two Ways to Use God's Whole Food Resources

Recipe: **MINUTE BRAN MUFFINS**[a] *Makes 10 muffins*		
Basic Ingredients	American Diet Choice	*Eating Better Lifestyle* Choice
Wheat bran	1½ cups bran cereal	1½ cups unprocessed
Flour	1½ cups all-purpose	1½ cups whole wheat
Sugar	1 cup brown sugar	⅓ cup honey
Fat	½ cup shortening	
Egg	1	1
Buttermilk	1 cup	1 cup
Soda	1¼ teaspoons	1¼ teaspoons
Salt	1¼ teaspoons	1 teaspoon
NUTRITION RESULTS (per muffin of 10)		
Basic Ingredients	American Diet Choice	*Eating Better Lifestyle* Choice
Calories	279	144
Protein	4.3 grams	4.9 grams
Fat	11.5 grams	1.6 grams
% of Calories in fat	35%	9%
Vitamins/ minerals[b]	70% less in flour[b]	70% more in flour
Dietary fiber	3.4 grams	5 grams
Sugar	6.3 teaspoons	1.6 teaspoons
Sodium	461 milligrams	350 milligrams
Cost[c]	$.18	$.13

---

a See the recipe section, p. 356, for this recipe.
b See "Total average loss," of 21 nutrients, p. 46.
c Cost based on average food costs, December 1994.

9

Eating Better Lifestyle Alternatives

———— ♥ ————

The man who eats everything must not look down on him who does not, and the man who does not eat everything must not condemn the man who does, for God has accepted him.

Romans 14:3

———— ♥ ————

*R*omans 14 teaches that there is more than one way to eat and that people ought not to judge one another for choosing different ways. Romans 14 does not teach that it doesn't matter what we eat. There are several criteria for making proper choices of food in Romans 14. For example Romans 14:5 says that "Each one should be fully convinced in his own mind." That guideline suggests that some intelligent forethought should be given to choices of food. Romans 14:23 teaches that what we eat should be a matter of faith. Mature Christian faith should be based on facts that reflect God's character and purpose rather than merely one's cultural tradition or personal tastes.

At this time there is much new and conflicting teaching about what is the most healthy way to eat. Nutrition certainly falls in the category of "disputable matters" (Romans 14:1). We need to be patient with both the situation and with others who choose different plans of eating. We believe there is adequate scriptural and scientific grounds for encouraging a change to the *Eating Better Lifestyle,* and also for defining what that lifestyle is. But there are several alternative dietary patterns that the *Eating Better Lifestyle* can adjust itself to. These include: 1) The Unlimited Plan; 2) The Lacto-Vegetarian Plan; 3) The Vegan Vegetarian Plan; 4) The No-Dairy, No-Egg Plan; 5) The Limited Food Combination Plan; 6) The Low Sodium Plan; 7) The Extra-Low-Fat Plan; and 8) The Therapeutic Diet Plan. We do not claim that these are the only diet plans, but they are the ones that have drawn the broadest attention among Americans, and they are the ones that we want to define in this book.

These alternatives may be briefly described as follows:

1) *The Unlimited Plan* does not exclude any major food groups. Meats, dairy products, fruits, vegetables, grains, beans, nuts, seeds, and natural sugars are all included. We have included an unlimited meal plan for dinner in Part 6.

2) *The Lacto-Vegetarian Plan* includes dairy products and sometimes eggs, and excludes meat, fish, and poultry. Part 6 includes a Lacto-Ovo-Vegetarian Meal Plan for dinners adaptable to a Lacto-Vegetarian Plan with minor adjustments.

3) *The Vegan Vegetarian Plan* includes plant foods only— no eggs, no dairy products, no meat, fish, or poultry. Care must be taken when following the vegan diet to get enough calcium and vitamin B_{12}. The best plant sources of calcium are broccoli and dark, leafy green vegetables. B_{12} can be supplied through seaweed or supplements. Several of our recipes are suitable for the vegan menu. A meal plan for 30

vegan vegetarian dinner menus is available in *Eating Better Main Dishes* (see p. 384).

4) *The No-Dairy, No-Egg Plan* includes meats, fish, and poultry but excludes eggs and dairy products. Part 7 includes a No-Dairy, No-Egg meal plan for dinners.

5) *The Limited Food Combinations Plan* follows several rules of combining foods but in essence they are: a) Eat fruits alone; b) Eat starchy carbohydrates with vegetables; c) Eat proteins with vegetables. Other combinations are not recommended. Several of the recipes in Part 7 are suitable for this plan. A meal plan for 39 limited food combination menus for dinners is given in *Eating Better Main Dishes* (see p. 384).

6) *The Low Sodium Plan* requires that all salt additions must be omitted from food. The Recommended Daily Allowance of sodium is 2400 milligrams. The average of menus in Part 6 are within the RDA limit. Salt may be omitted from the recipes, but we do not recommend it as this significantly affects the taste appeal. Most people do not need a severely restricted salt diet (see chapter 25). Of all the diet plans, we think this one is the least important and the least appealing.

7) *The Extra-Low-Fat Plan* limits fat intake to 20% or less of calories. Menus in Part 7 are 23% fat. Fourteen of our menus are 20% fat or less. *Eating Better Main Dishes* provides a meal plan with 61 extra-low-fat menus (see p. 384).

8) *The Therapeutic Diet Plan* is any diet plan that is more or less tailor-made for an individual with specific health problems. Most of the recipes in Part 7 are easily adaptable for use in therapeutic diets.

It is our desire to make the *Eating Better Lifestyle* as flexible and useful to as many needs, tastes, interests, and nutritional convictions that we can. It is a very flexible eating lifestyle. Also, you may be assured that each one of these alternatives, with good planning, will provide adequate nutrition. Restrictions aside, they are all superior in health benefits to the American Diet.

PART 3

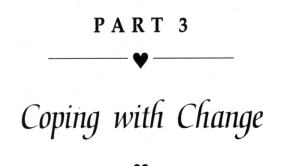

Coping with Change

10

First Things First

---- ♥ ----

Have I not commanded you? Be strong and coura-
geous. Do not be terrified; do not be discouraged, for the
LORD your God will be with you wherever you go.

Joshua 1:9

---- ♥ ----

*W*hen the Israelites had crossed the Red Sea, Moses
sent 12 men into Canaan to survey the land and
bring back some of its abundant fresh produce. Only two of
the men, Joshua and Caleb, returned with the optimistic
report that they could conquer the land. The remaining ten
men saw only the strong fortified cities filled with powerful people (Numbers 13). The difference between their fear
and Joshua's and Caleb's confidence was the faith that God
had already promised to give them the land. Would God
give such a promise without providing His presence and
strength to fulfill it?

The fear of changing our eating lifestyle is a legitimate
one considering that almost everything needs to be totally
overhauled! So much is involved—the taste preferences of

everyone we feed, finding new shopping resources, developing new food preparation skills, new menu planning, new food storage methods, new food budgeting, and new recipes.

God commanded Joshua to be strong and unafraid because his task was God-given. The first step in making the *Eating Better Lifestyle* change is commitment to the Lord, for, "it is the Lord Christ you are serving" (Colossians 3:24).

Next, develop the *Eating Better Lifestyle* one step at a time. Don't try to do everything at once. Note how Moses sent the men to survey the land before launching campaigns to conquer it (Numbers 13). Use the whys and how-tos of this book to plan your own strategy and time schedule. Don't judge your progress by someone else's standard. Concentrate on making the basic changes first.

The meal plans, menus, recipes, suggestions for improving your own favorite recipes, and guidelines for dining out in Part 6 reflect the following basic changes:

> *more fiber*: include more whole grains, dry beans, fresh fruits, and fresh vegetables
>
> *more vitamins and minerals*: same as above
>
> *less fat*: reduce red meats, reduce use of vegetable oils, margarine, butter, and shortening in cooking and in packaged foods; add more fiber as above; use more of the nonfat and low-fat dairy products and cheeses
>
> *less refined sugar*: cut amount by half—use honey in place of sugar; omit canned and packaged foods with sugar
>
> *less sodium*: leave salt off the table; reduce canned and packaged food items that contain salt; do not add salt to vegetables
>
> *controlled calories*: all of the above will contribute wonderfully—without counting!

Leave detailed refinements for later when you have begun to feel more comfortable with the *Eating Better Lifestyle*. For example, arrowroot powder is more nutritious than cornstarch, but it is a minor ingredient in comparison to white flour versus whole-grain flour. For another example, choosing organically grown produce* has merit, but choosing more fresh fruits and vegetables of any kind is more important. The point is, major on the majors.

---

* See definition, p. 187.

11

Overcoming the Four Fears:
What About Taste?

───── ♥ ─────

If you falter in times of trouble, how small is your strength!

Proverbs 24:10

I can do everything through him who gives me strength.

Philippians 4:13

───── ♥ ─────

*P*eople considering the *Eating Better Lifestyle* face four fears: 1) "I am afraid it won't taste good"; 2) "I am afraid it will take too much time"; 3) "I am afraid it will cost too much"; and 4) "I am afraid it will be too difficult to find the ingredients."

───── ♥ ─────

Appealing taste is the single most important reason why we choose to eat what we do. People often give other excuses for not changing their eating patterns when the real reason is fear of unfamiliar taste. Sue's technically oriented friend Bob, a California Institute of Technology graduate, thought that he needed all the nutrient data to prove the value of whole foods first. That was true until he ate our four-grain pancakes! He loved them. It was the satisfaction of that taste which motivated him to change his eating habits.

The frequent criticism of health food is that it does not taste good. We agree. Why? One reason is that too many health enthusiasts become too restrictive in their choices of ingredients and recipes. Some leave all the salt and all the fat out of recipes. The result is bland and blah food. It takes real skill to find other seasonings to compensate. Another problem is that many health-food advocates expect people to adopt a menu and recipe pattern that is not American— no more hamburgers, no more pizza, no more meat and potatoes. Our recipes are certainly not all hamburgers and pizza, but they retain the familiar American tastes. Katherine's comment reflects a typical response: "My family has enjoyed the food I've cooked from your books. I feel a peaceful balance in our eating and don't feel so frustrated in my attempts to provide good nutrition."

We'd like to share our secret of how to develop good-tasting recipes. Here are some simple guidelines. First, start with recipes and menus familiar to your family's tastes but improve the nutritional quality of some of the ingredients. For example, instead of cutting hamburgers out of the menu, use meat that is lower in fat such as ground turkey. Then put it on whole-wheat hamburger buns instead of white bread buns. Check out Part 6 for more ideas on this. Second, read the salt and fat chapters to see why you don't have to cut all the salt and fat out of recipes. Indeed you ought not cut out all the fat! Third, change those things first that your tastes can handle. So tofu and brown rice don't appeal to you now—try whole-wheat spaghetti instead. If you aren't ready for whole-wheat flour, try half whole-wheat and half white flour.

Finally, be patient with yourself and those you serve. Remember: The objective is to win the war, not just a little skirmish. Experiment with new recipes. Don't expect everyone to like everything. It may take two years before you hear the words that one young mother finally heard from her once-skeptical husband, "Dear, I want you to try every recipe in that book!" We can assure you that our *Eating Better Lifestyle* recipes have an excellent track record of family appeal. One lady stated it well: "You use 'real people' food but it's done in a healthy way." And Teri wrote, "We have sure enjoyed the recipes. All health food is not blah, we've found."

God has created enough variety for you to select what appeals to your family. Trust the One who created taste buds for His whole foods to give you skill and wisdom in choosing and timing your presentations of new dishes.

The white flour and brown sugar cinnamon rolls that Sue once baked for summer campers on Catalina Island were the highlight of each week's breakfasts. Later after she learned to bake cinnamon rolls with honey and whole-wheat flour for her family, they returned to camp. They discovered that the white flour, refined sugar cinnamon rolls didn't provide the satisfaction they had learned to enjoy in the whole-grain-and-honey version, and they realized then that their taste buds could, indeed, adapt to enjoy the flavors and textures of food for which they were created.

They use a family rating scale to evaluate the taste of new recipes (p. 78). It can be a real help in assisting the transition. To assure your success, we've put taste as the first priority in selecting the recipes and menus in Part 7.

12

Overcoming the Four Fears:
What About Time?

———— ♥ ————

There is a time for everything, and a season for every activity under heaven.

Ecclesiastes 3:1

———— ♥ ————

*F*ast-food outlets, TV dinners, prepackaged foods, and the microwave oven are rapidly producing a generation of noncooks. Lack of time has become a real obstacle to quality home food preparation because there are so many alternatives to cooking. Indeed, even the lovely tray of fresh fruit or vegetable platter with dip brought to the church potluck may just as well have come from Smith's Supermarket, or that basket of yummy blueberry muffins from Costco. Nothing is left undone—even the salad is made. Just pick it up on the way to the potluck and set it on the table. But does developing the *Eating Better Lifestyle* now mean that we must spend hours slaving in our kitchens? No!

No one has been given more than 24 hours for each day. The secret is not to get more time. It is to manage our time. It takes only a little time to plan the saving of much time. This is the purpose of Emilie's More Hours in My Day seminars. During the initial period of transition, the *Eating Better Lifestyle* requires careful planning. That is why we have included a section in Part 6 on how to do it. In addition, more help is available beyond what we have covered in this book (pp. 379-381).

Save the more complex recipes for later. Start with supermarket ingredients that require very simple preparation such as *Brown Rice* (p. 312) or *Lentil Rice Casserole* (p. 315). Many prepackaged whole-food items of nutritional quality are now available. Just remember to read the ingredients label (see chapter 54)!

Use your freezer to save time. Prepare freezer main dishes. Set aside a period of time when you are most relaxed and free of other chores to prepare several dishes for the freezer at a time. You do not need to set aside an entire day for this, nor do you need to prepare an entire month of meals all at once. In just two to four hours you can easily prepare four to five main dishes for the freezer. *Eating Better Casseroles* (see p. 384 for information) provides 26 delicious meals with a grocery list and assembly order for preparing five casseroles at a time, plus a menu suggestion for each casserole. In addition, *Eating Better Casseroles* includes 20 "Extra Timesaving Tips," many of them utilizing the freezer. *Meals in Minutes* (Harvest House Publishers) provides nine sets of three casseroles, each with a grocery list, assembly list, and menu suggestions, plus 20 other quick *Eating Better* meals with menu suggestions. *Meals in Minutes* also introduces you to four 3-in-1 cooking plans, making the freezer method very flexible and easy for different interests and needs. If you do not own a freezer, freezer meals are worth buying one for! You will be amazed at how quickly your freezer will fill up with tasty made-in-advance dishes once you embark on an easy plan that suits your own busy schedule.

Becky, a home-schooling mother of six boys, ages 3–11, decided to give the freezer casseroles a try. She reported, "I modified the plan and cooked about 4–5 times as much each night for eight days. We are about two weeks into the frozen dinners and I love it. It has helped my home management immensely. I have gotten so much more done this last week, like correspondence and mending—things that I rarely get done."

Besides saving you many hours of time, the freezer will facilitate putting foods of higher nutritional quality at less cost on your table. Our *Eating Better* freezer main dishes and casseroles average 40% less fat, 40% less cholesterol, 40% less sodium, and 220% more dietary fiber than typical American dishes, and at a 25% lower cost. The dollar savings over commercial pre-prepared meals is even higher, not to mention that your own freezer meals have that wonderful home-cooked taste appeal that commercial offerings seldom can match. About a year after Becky started to freeze casseroles, she was diagnosed with multiple sclerosis. When asked by the ladies in her church what they could do to help her, she requested them to meet her in the church kitchen to prepare a month of freezer meals for her family. She has been able to use many of our frozen casseroles with slight modifications for her specialized diet. Being on a strict budget, she appreciates the cost savings.

Your freezer will reduce the frequency of your shopping trips, as well, especially to health-food stores that may be further away from you than the local supermarket. Even though Sue has access to three supermarkets within three-fourths of a mile of her home, her favorite multigrain bread (ten grains plus two legumes) comes from a store 20 miles away. When on business trips in the area, she stops and purchases several loaves at a time to put in the freezer. Thus, if you do not have time for home baking, you can still have various kinds of whole-grain breads, rolls, and buns on hand right from your freezer.

Quick breads with light batters such as waffles, pancakes, muffins, coffee cakes, crepes, and popovers can be prepared quickly in the blender starting with unmilled whole grains. We call this "blender batter baking"—a revolutionary concept in quick preparation with the freshest grain possible without owning a grain mill. Several recipes for all of these quick breads are available in **Breakfasts** (see p. 384). Try our *Minute Blender Bran Muffins, 5-Minute Blender Waffles or Pancakes, and Whole-Wheat Popovers* in the blender (see recipe section).

Many women have inquired about making whole-grain yeast breads in the automatic bread-making machines that do everything for you from start to finish after you have put in the ingredients. Our experience has been, so far, that producing an all-whole-grain loaf of truly acceptable texture is a tricky business. Most women resort to using some refined white bread flour for improved texture. Some companies that manufacture the bread machines are seeking ways to improve their machines for all-whole-grain breads, and cookbooks that address this issue are appearing in bookstores. The all-whole-grain bread recipes in George Burnett's *The Breadman's Healthy Bread Book* look delicious, though we have not tried them. The automatic bread machine has ushered in a new era of technology that will match the precise performance of specific machines with specific recipes. Emilie and I prefer making yeast breads with our Bosch Kitchen Machines. Many women also make breads in the DLX Kitchen Machine, a product of Magic Mill (there are many dealers throughout the country). Both of these machines are very "forgiving" of recipes not tailor-made for them. They consistently turn out terrific bread, requiring only about 10 to 15 minutes of your time to make 4 to 10 loaves of bread, although they are not fully automatic and will not shape loaves and bake them for you.

Some food preparation steps can be omitted for nutritional reasons. You can omit peeling carrots and potatoes, for example, and benefit from the additional nutrients and fiber (see exception to peeling potatoes, p. 154). We have even reduced our cooking of vegetables, opting to eat them raw. Instead of a small salad with an additional cooked vegetable, we frequently eat a large tossed salad with more raw vegetables. A great last-minute time-saver is to clean and dry your salad greens in advance. A very quick and effective method is outlined in *Meals in Minutes* on p. 155 (*Lettuce Wash 'n Dry!*) and in *Survival for Busy Women* on p. 88 (see p. 383 for information). For effective ways to clean fruits and vegetables that will be eaten unpeeled, see p. 153.

Don't forget to include your children in food preparation. If they fix it, they will eat it. Little hands may be messy now, but they can become time-savers for you later when they plan the menus, do the shopping, and prepare some of the meals (as our children in their teens have done). As they become independent young adults, they will leave home with valuable survival skills.

Taking time to plan the family food strategy is part of our God-given role. Food manufacturers and merchandizers would like to get us to pay them to do it for us. Part of their persuasive tactic is to convince us that unpaid, unrecognized service is also unworthy. Not so with Jesus. For example, in Luke 8:2,3 a group of women (much better off financially) followed Jesus and His disciples and provided for their physical needs. This freed Jesus to give His time to preaching and healing. In Acts 6:1-7 the apostles appointed men with the highest spiritual qualifications for the service of food distribution: "We will turn this responsibility over to them and will give our attention to prayer and the ministry of the word" (verses 3,4). Not only is providing food a necessary task, it is worthy of godly attention by some people in order to free others to carry out the work God has given them to do.

13

Overcoming the Four Fears:
What About Cost?

———— ♥ ————

*Why spend money on what is not bread, and your labor
on what does not satisfy? Listen, listen to me, and eat
what is good, and your soul will delight in the richest of
fare.*

Isaiah 55:2

———— ♥ ————

*L*osing one's health is a costly ordeal. Rising health-
care costs are a focus of deep concern in the 1990s. In
addition to medical costs, the cost of days of work lost
through illness runs in the millions. In fact, some corporations have fitness programs for employees. These programs
are proving to be less costly than the employee days of
work lost. These businesses are learning that preventive
measures to maintain health are an economic benefit. Preventive health care is becoming more necessary than ever
for survival. If mandated universal health care paid for by

taxes becomes a reality in America, medical services to the very young and the elderly in particular, and medical services to all in general, may be curbed or rationed. We must do all that we can for ourselves to maintain our health.

Good nutrition is an economical preventive health-care measure. Eating nutritionally inferior food saves neither money nor life. Such foods fill the stomach but fail to satisfy the real nutrient needs of the body. Jamie discovered this with her son, Tim. Tim missed 47 days of school and spent seven-and-a-half days in the hospital in the second and third grade. His medical costs were over $1,000 for one year. Jamie's family began the *Eating Better Lifestyle* as Tim entered the fourth grade. In the three years that followed Tim missed five days of school and there were no medical expenses!

The USDA issues quarterly reports of changes in individual and family food costs for eating at home. They are divided into four categories: thrifty, low budget, moderate budget, and liberal. We should note, however, that the amount spent does not reflect the difference between a poor diet or a good diet.

Where we eat makes a great difference as to what food costs. By 1983 Americans were eating 42% of their meals in restaurants. In 1984 Americans spent $1,800 per person in fast-food restaurants,[1] an average of almost $5.00 per day— higher than the liberal budget food plan of eating at home in 1986. This trend has continued into the 1990s. Usually we will find enough money to buy what we consider important. Certainly, we can trust our God to give us the wisdom to spend wisely for good nutrition what money we do have for food.

While some *Eating Better Lifestyle* foods are more costly item for item, the overall cost may be less expensive. Note the cost, for example, of *Minute Blender Bran Muffins* (p. 356). Our muffins are less expensive than typical American muffins. While the whole-wheat flour and the honey are more expensive ingredients than white flour and white sugar, the unprocessed bran is less expensive than bran cereal, and shortening—a costly ingredient—is not used in the more nutritious muffins.

We also significantly shift the expense of the food bill when we purchase smaller amounts of high-fat, high-protein foods such as meats and dairy products. This gives us more dollars to spend on some of the more nutritious food items such as whole grains and fresh vegetables. These can be combined in delicious recipes with herbs for flavoring and a little meat added. The end result is a menu that is less costly than the menu using a prepackaged refined-food item and a larger meat serving. Sue has made extensive comparisons between *Eating Better* menus and typical American meals. Our meals average 25% less in cost. An even greater savings can be realized utilizing our 52 extra-low-budget meals from **Main Dishes** and soup and muffin menus from **Soups & Muffins** at an average cost of $1.20 per adult serving. This is 35% below the typical American budget dinner of $1.85 (as of January 1995, based on a 3% yearly increase in food prices since June 1989). The average cost of our 37 menus in the recipe section, as of January 1995, will be $1.76—below the average cost of typical American budget dinners. Of those 37 menus, 28 are $1.85 or lower. Only two menus are over $2.00 and only two menus are over $3.00. One lady wrote, "A big thank-you for taking everyday stuff and making it appealing to our budget as well as our palates." Another wrote, "My groceries are now running between $100 to $115 a week instead of $125 to $135." She was realizing a 15% to 20% savings. That eating "health food" must necessarily cost more is a myth.

When considering the real expense of food, we must think in terms of value received for dollars spent. Refined prepackaged foods will always cost more than basic food staples. You will always pay for the labor of pre-prepared food, its fancy packaging to attract your attention, and the advertising to encourage you to buy it. Basic food staples such as grains, dry beans, fresh fruits, and vegetables get little advertising promotion, are not generally put into fancy packaging, and require little pre-preparation. More of your food dollar is therefore being spent on the nutritional value.

There are many ways to economize the food budget without sacrificing nutritional value. Here are several. Even if you choose to do only one or two of them, you will realize a significant savings:

- ♥ Bake whole-grain breads rather than buy them.
- ♥ Grow, rather than buy, sprouts.
- ♥ Grow as much as you can in your own garden— feed the soil with your food scraps for a rich growing medium instead of feeding them to the disposal or garbage can. Have a covered container conveniently located in the kitchen in which to put your food scraps—empty it once a day into your outdoor compost heap.
- ♥ Take advantage of in-season fruits and vegetables.
- ♥ Take advantage of sales on nutritious basic food items.
- ♥ Reduce the number of desserts in your menu.
- ♥ Participate in a food co-op.
- ♥ Utilize leftovers wisely.
- ♥ Plan your menus.
- ♥ Shop only from a planned grocery list.
- ♥ Minimize your shopping trips.
- ♥ Purchase nonperishable food items or items that keep well in the freezer in quantity or economy sizes (a freezer is a wise economy investment, especially for the single person who uses smaller amounts of many perishable items).
- ♥ Limit visits to restaurants and fast-food outlets. Share meals.

- ♥ Don't buy every "health food" alternative for every "junk food" available (such as cookies, candy, etc.).

- ♥ Use meats more frequently in small amounts as a supplement to dinner menus rather than as the main food item.

- ♥ Have several "meatless" meals during the week.

- ♥ Develop the habit of drinking more water in place of juices, fruit beverages, pop, coffee, etc.

- ♥ Fast one day a week and save $$! (See chapter 45.)

- ♥ Buy grains and beans—the least-expensive food items.

The person committed to nutritional quality as a standard for life and health will find ways to make the food budget work. An example is our friend, Loretta. For several years Loretta, mother of eight children ages 4 to 18 years, lived as a single parent in low-income housing, alternating between low-paying jobs and welfare. Yet, because she was committed to the value of good nutrition for her family, she maintained the *Eating Better Lifestyle* for many years, even during lean periods such as the last week of the month when there was no money left. If there was only enough to purchase an economy sack of potatoes, she would feed the family potatoes for a week. Loretta even purchased a home flour mill. Baking her own bread instead of purchasing 14 loaves a week brought considerable savings, and her family has eaten many a whole-grain pancake!

14

Overcoming the Four Fears:
What About Resources?

———— ♥ ————

She is like the merchant ships, bringing her food from afar.

Proverbs 31:14

———— ♥ ————

*A*vailability of fresh fruits and vegetables varies widely by season and by where you live. Certain staples, however, are available almost anywhere there is a market demand. Most supermarkets will carry brown rice, dry beans and peas, fresh fruits and vegetables, buttermilk, yogurt, lowfat milk, chicken, fish, turkey, cheddar and mozzarella cheese, whole-wheat flour, rolled oats, unprocessed bran, raisins, dates, honey, peanut butter without sugar or hydrogenated fat, nuts and seeds, olive oil, soy sauce, unsweetened canned pineapple and applesauce, frozen vegetables, and herbs and spices. These items can help you to get a good start. Start reading labels (p. 294) in order to choose the most nutritious food items available. An excellent resource for supermarket purchasing of whole-food items and brands in different areas of the country is *The Supermarket Handbook* by Nikki and David Goldbeck. We have also given some mail-order resources (pp. 290-92).

Don't hesitate to request your local supermarket manager to carry whole-food items such as ground turkey and whole-grain breads, for example. Don't be passive about it. Markets are created by customer needs, and businesses always want to profit from those needs that rise to the level of demands. Read the labels to find the best available and then request something better, if needed. Sometimes it is easy to overlook what we don't expect to find. For example, Sue's friend Jan, who lives in Washington, D.C., asked us for suggestions where she might purchase whole grains. While visiting her, Sue went shopping one morning at the local supermarket where Jan always shops. There were large bins full of several whole grains and beans. She had just never thought to look for them there! There are wholesome food items in supermarkets, and the number will continue to increase as awareness of good nutrition grows.

For other resources check the many categories in the phone book yellow pages that we have listed on page 303. The quality and offerings of health food stores vary widely from vitamin pill shops to exotic herb importers, from the archaic to the leaders in the whole-foods industry. Go with the ingredient checklist (pp. 272-75) in hand just to check out what is available. Ask questions. Sue sends her cooking class students with a three-page list. It sometimes creates quite a stir! Many health-food store owners specialize in obtaining items unavailable in the supermarkets. Some will special order items in bulk at lower prices. Be aggressive. If we have told you about an ingredient, it's available. In Sue's *Eating Better* recipes she lists a reference page number right next to each unfamiliar ingredient so that you can turn right to the page that tells you what the ingredient is and where to purchase it. We have carried out this idea in the recipe section of this book (see an example of this on p. 308).

A food co-op can provide good variety at wholesale prices. Co-ops range in sophistication from those which are a simple ministry to a few friends and neighbors to large organizations. In a co-op several people pool their orders to gain the advantage of bulk prices. Co-ops work best when a group of people with a common need who know each other on a face-to-face basis follow agreed-upon rules that assure equitable rewards for all.

While we suggest you purchase the most nutritious form of some ingredients, such as low-sodium baking powder, sea salt, and less refined oils that are available only in health-food stores, recipes may be prepared without them. It is better to start with what you have than not start at all.

15

Helping My Family to Change

---- ♥ ----

She speaks with wisdom, and faithful instruction is on her tongue. She watches over the affairs of her household and does not eat the bread of idleness. Her children arise and call her blessed; her husband also, and he praises her.

Proverbs 31:26-28

---- ♥ ----

*W*hatever our individual dietary needs may be, most of us must provide food for a family. Short-order cooking for individual tastes and needs is impractical and time-consuming. Therefore, making the change to the *Eating Better Lifestyle* realistically needs to become a family affair. We have several additional suggestions for helping your family to change in this chapter, but actually many of the things that help to motivate you personally can help to motivate your family as well. Sharing these things in a spirit of love, gentleness, and understanding in a way appropriate to the various ages and temperaments of family members will do a lot to gain acceptance. Pray for the love of Jesus Christ to come through you to your family, because it is as the Holy Spirit changes the heart and renews the mind of each person that true change comes.

If you are married, discuss your desire to make changes with your husband before you start. Pray for wisdom about how to do this, keeping his temperament in mind. If you are not familiar with temperament types, you will find Florence Littauer's books—*Your Personality Tree, Personality Plus,* or *How to Get Along With Difficult People*—helpful. While the books do not address food issues specifically, it is very easy to understand that different temperaments will respond differently to food change. If your husband is phlegmatic, for example, he may not get very excited about your adventure, but he will probably be willing to go along with it. If he wants to be more involved in the decision making, cooperate with him and be willing to consider possible limitations to what you can do. If he or any other family member is not like-minded with you, pray for a change of heart and attitudes.

What you can explain to children depends on their ages, but practically all children from a very young age have a natural curiosity and keen interest in taking part in food planning and preparation. Our *"Eating Better with Sue"* video cooking course and **Lunches & Snacks with Lessons for Children** are excellent teaching resources from age eight to adult. **Lunches & Snacks** includes a chart showing what you can expect children to learn at different ages, starting at age two. Our lessons for children focus on kid-pleasing recipes accompanied by a "nutrition quiz" for informal family discussion while making and eating the recipe (see, for example, p. 364 in the recipe section). All the nutrition answers you need are provided in the lessons. You do not need to be a nutrition expert.

You have a wonderful opportunity to make the adventure of new foods a part of learning together. Be willing to see what food change means through the eyes of each one. For example, the sanguine child wants to have fun and thrives on compliments. If you have such a child, you might explore what food activities he/she would especially have fun doing. Maybe it is shopping with you, or maybe it is baking cookies. Capitalize on these interests and then freely compliment the child for his/her efforts. The choleric child, the melancholy child, the phlegmatic child, or children with combinations of temperament will react differently from the sanguine.

All family members will want to feel that you care about their reactions to new foods and recipes. Taste enjoyment will be their number-one concern. Sue's family uses a rating scale of 1 to 10 to evaluate each new dish. A rating of 1 means, "Let's please not repeat this one!" A rating of 10 means, "This is really tasty. Let's have it often." A rating anywhere in between gives Sue some indication whether she can improve the recipe by altering some of the ingredients, and how often to serve it. In most cases, if the recipe does not rate an 8 or higher after ingredient adjustments are made, it does not become a part of Sue's recipe file. This one activity of using the rating scale accomplishes several things: 1) It fulfills each person's need to know that his/her opinion matters. 2) It gives Sue an organized plan for building a new recipe file that everyone will enjoy. 3) It takes the pressure off the cook because we all agree that we are not rating the cook's ability, but the recipe. 4) Complaining is minimized because there is assurance that if a recipe is not tasty, it will not become a future part of family meals. If one or two do not like what everyone else agrees is tasty, Sue will make an effort to serve other food with it next time for those who don't care for it. 5) It conveys the idea that this is a family project and that we are experimenting together. When using a rating scale it is a good idea to ask such questions as, "How do you like the taste—is it too bland, too spicy?" "How do you like the texture—the feel of it in your mouth?" "How do you like the smell?" "How does it look to you—is it attractive, colorful?" Keep the perspective that change to better eating is the goal.

Include a special night at least once a month when you serve each person's favorite meal or recipe, improving the nutritional quality of some of the ingredients where you can. If changes don't work well, don't take away the dish until other tasty, but more nutritious dishes, will compensate. You don't have to serve such favorites every day.

Establish some special snack/treat traditions. One mother told us she surprised her children with a small baggie of dates, nuts, and raisins she mixed herself. They thought that was special because she made it special. They didn't know about sugared treats. Another mom shared that her son likes carrot sticks as a treat. Emilie's mother would bake her a potato for an after-school snack. It was a treat and it became a special memory that Emilie passed on to her children. Often we miss the fact that such simple and plain food items give children special pleasure when given in the context of family love.

Mrs. Jones taught Sue to bake cookies (whole-grain with honey, of course) just before the children arrived home from school so that the lovely aroma greeted them as they walked in the door. Another welcome treat is a hot carob drink and/or popcorn waiting for the child who has just sloshed home through the pouring rain. You don't need to get into a rut with ordinary snacks. For example, cut out your 100% whole-wheat bread with a heart shape, teddy bear, rabbit, or Mickey Mouse cookie cutter. Spread a favorite topping on it such as peanut butter or a light covering of honey-butter. Use raisins as eyes, nose, and mouth. Kids will love it! Take a lesson from television food advertising. Big food companies capture our imagination with clever ideas to promote their products. Let's use our imaginations to advertise our own healthy foods!

Your family will be influenced more by your attitude than by your nutritional pronouncements. It is better not to label your new dishes as "health food," "macrobiotic," or "vegetarian." Avoid a situation where food choices become a battle of the wills. Love changes people, but force seldom does. Here are some Scriptures that will give you real support:

Cheerful attitude—Proverbs 17:22

Don't nag—Proverbs 15:1,17; Proverbs 17:1,14; Proverbs 21:23; Philippians 2:14

Apply fruit of the Spirit—Galatians 5:22,23

Take authority over children—Proverbs 22:6,15; Ephesians 6:1

Speak truth in love—Ephesians 4:15

Gentle and quiet spirit—1 Peter 3:4; Philippians 4:5

Not anxious, but prayerful—Philippians 4:6,7

Right motives—1 Thessalonians 1:3; 1 Corinthians 13:13

Hopefulness—Proverbs 23:18

PART 4

———— ♥ ————

Nitty Gritty
Nutrition News

———— ♥ ————

16

Food Mythology Quiz

——— ♥ ———

It is the glory of God to conceal a matter; to search out a matter is the glory of kings.

Proverbs 25:2

——— ♥ ———

Circle T for True, F for False:

T F   Vitamin-mineral supplements will make up for the nutrition that is lacking in the food I eat.

T F   If I quit eating meat I won't get enough protein.

T F   I must use dairy products if I expect to get enough calcium.

T F   Carbohydrates are fattening.

T F   Fat is fattening.

T F   Salt is bad for your health.

T F   Honey is no better than sugar.

T F   Margarine is healthier than butter.

T   F   Cholesterol is bad for your health.

T   F   Raw milk is dangerous.

T   F   Cooked food is dead food.

T   F   To lose weight, eat fewer calories.

T   F   If it's "natural," it's good for you.

All of these statements reflect popular beliefs about food. In the following chapters we will discuss these issues so you can make wiser food choices.

17

Nutrients on Parade

———— ♥ ————

———— ♥ ————

*I*n addition to oxygen and water the human body needs five groups of known nutrients: carbohydrates, protein, fats, vitamins, and minerals. The first three are called macronutrients and the last two are called micronutrients. We can sort them out easily in the following chart:

Macronutrients: The body uses larger amounts measured in grams. These groups have energy value.

　　—Carbohydrates:　　1 gram = 4 calories
　　—Protein:　　　　　1 gram = 4 calories
　　—Fats:　　　　　　 1 gram = 9 calories

Micronutrients: The body uses smaller amounts measured in International Units, milligrams, or micrograms (I.U., mg., mcg.). These groups have no energy value (meaning no calories).

—Vitamins: about 20 known vitamins
—Minerals: about 17 known minerals

The body needs about 40 known nutrients.

Carbohydrates, fats, proteins, and water are the substances that food is made of in varying combinations. Vitamins and minerals are contained within the carbohydrates, fats, and proteins. Water contains minerals. All of these nutrients work synergistically in the body for health. The synergism of nutrients means that they work more effectively together than separately. For example, each body cell is like a small factory building the materials necessary for life. This process requires larger amounts of some nutrients and minute amounts of others. Yet every nutrient working together with the others is essential to the health of the whole. Therefore, it is difficult to talk about the functions of each nutrient in an isolated way as if it performed certain things all by itself. *The Nutrition Almanac* provides listings of what nutrients work synergistically together (see Recommended Reading, p. 381).

Another way to explain synergism is by Paul's analogy of the human body to the Body of Christ. "Now the body is not made up of one part but of many. . . . The eye cannot say to the hand, 'I don't need you!' And the head cannot say to the feet, 'I don't need you!' . . . If one part suffers, every part suffers with it; if one part is honored, every part rejoices with it" (1 Corinthians 12:14,21,26). Of course, we know that a body can live and function without a hand, an eye, or a foot, but it cannot survive without the head or heart. So it is with food nutrients. Nutrient deficiencies can lead to severe health problems, increased susceptibility to infectious diseases, degenerative diseases, and eventually death. Although we discuss each nutrient group separately for simplicity in the following chapters, we do not want to lose sight of the whole. Each nutrient performs its job fully only in the presence of all the other nutrients supplied in adequate amounts.

Simply stated, God has stored all these nutrients together in a wonderful whole-food variety pack!

18

The Challenge of Carbohydrates

———— ♥ ————

Awk! I can't eat a high-carbohydrate diet! I'll get fat!"

———— ♥ ————

Yes, that's right—bread, pastas, cakes, cookies, chips, and candy are fattening! Everybody who's on a diet knows that these foods are out! So carbohydrates must be fattening, right? Wrong! In general, most Americans fail to appreciate carbohydrates because they are confused about what carbohydrates really are.

Carbohydrates are classified in two groups:

1) *simple carbohydrates*:
   sugars present in fruits, honey, maple syrup, sugar cane
   —quick, high-energy foods

2) *complex carbohydrates*:
   starches and dietary fibers present in whole grains, beans and peas, starchy vegetables (potatoes, squash), nuts and seeds
   —slow-releasing, high-energy foods
   —dietary fibers and pure water in fresh fruits and vegetables
   —low-energy, cleansing foods

But carbohydrates may also be classified in another way:

1) *unrefined carbohydrates*:
   fresh fruits, fresh vegetables, whole grains, beans and peas, naturally occurring sugars (e.g. honey), nuts and seeds

2) *refined carbohydrates*:
   carbohydrate foods stripped of dietary fiber, vitamins, and minerals through processing (e.g. white sugar, white flour, prepackaged foods and mixes made with white sugar and white flour, white rice, degerminated corn-meal, sugary canned fruits and juice)

The entire list—breads, pastas, cakes, cookies, chips, and candy—makes up 50% of our diet in the refined carbohydrate form. We love them, and we know they are addictive and make us fat! No wonder we are confused about the nutritional value of carbohydrates!

God's design for carbohydrates is much different. He planned them to be our primary source of energy for all the body processes, assistants in metabolizing protein and fat, reservoirs of pure water, wonderful sources of satiating, digestive and fat-regulating fibers, and gold mines of essential vitamins and minerals. These are carbohydrates as man once knew them, and they are the first foods God gave us in the beginning of creation: "I give you every seed-bearing plant on the face of the whole earth and every tree

that has fruit with seed in it. They will be yours for food"
(Genesis 1:29). Unrefined carbohydrates are the core of the
Eating Better Lifestyle. They include both the higher-calorie
starches and the lower-calorie fruits and vegetables. They
all contain one nonfattening treasure—dietary fiber.

19

Making Friends with Fiber

———— ♥ ————

Great are the works of the LORD; they are pondered by all who delight in them.

Psalm 111:2

———— ♥ ————

*I*ncredible as it may seem, the lack of just one food nutrient—dietary fiber—contributes to tragic suffering in America. Millions are burdened by digestive disorders, cancers, heart disease, diabetes, and obesity. Fiber is a God-given resource. Remove it from our foods and we suffer.

Kinds of Fiber

Actually, fiber has not traditionally been classified as a nutrient. Part of the fiber in plant foods was discovered in 1887 and labeled as crude fiber. Many food package labels still listed only crude fiber through the 1980s. In 1972 dietary fiber was discovered. It includes several different types of fiber. There is three to seven times more dietary fiber than crude fiber in foods. The new labeling law now requires the listing of dietary fiber on all packaged foods (see chapter 58, "Nutrient Data and The New Labeling Law").

Dietary fiber includes water-soluble fibers and insoluble fibers. The water-soluble fibers are gums and pectins. The best food sources of gums are oats, especially the bran, and all beans and peas (legumes). The best sources of pectin are apples, citrus fruits, carrots, cauliflower, squash, green beans, cabbage, dried peas, strawberries, and potatoes. The insoluble fibers are cellulose, hemicelluloses, and lignin. The best sources of these fibers are whole grains including whole wheat, especially wheat bran. Apples, carrots, green and wax beans, peppers, cabbage, broccoli, brussels sprouts, and young peas are also excellent sources of cellulose. Mature vegetables, strawberries, eggplant, pears, green beans, and radishes are high in lignin. Most vegetables, grains, beans and peas, and nuts and seeds contain more than one dietary fiber in varying proportions. The amounts and effects of these fibers can vary with the stage of growth, the age of the plants, and the way the food is prepared.

Functions of Fiber

Dietary fibers perform different functions in the human body. Insoluble fibers add bulk by absorbing water in the digestive track. This speeds up the transit time of food through the digestive system. Lack of bulk contributes to constipation, hiatus hernia, gallstones, diverticulosis, spastic colon, hemorrhoids, varicose veins, diarrhea, colitis, appendicitis, and colon cancer. Insoluble fibers may also help to remove toxins, pesticide residues, and carcinogenic bacteria from the body.

Soluble fibers, and also lignin, help to regulate blood cholesterol and triglyceride levels, decrease fat absorption, and moderate wide swings in blood sugar levels. These processes are important for the prevention and moderation of hypoglycemia, diabetes, heart disease, and weight. The satiety value of fiber, the feeling of being full, also assists weight control. Fewer calories of high-fiber foods are more filling and also require more chewing. The "I've had enough" signals will reach the brain before you have overeaten. In addition "carbohydrate goes through different pathways from fat—pathways that burn off more calories."[1] Of course, we are talking about unrefined carbohydrate calories and not white sugar and white flour!

Considerable research lends support to these benefits. The British medical journal, *Lancet*, September 4, 1982, reported the findings of a ten-year Netherlands study performed on 871 men. The death rate among the men on low-fiber diets was four times higher from heart disease, three times higher from cancer, and three times higher from all causes than that of the men who ate about 37 grams of dietary fiber per day. Disease declined proportionately with the increase of dietary fiber. Studies of countries reveal that societies with high-fiber diets consistently have significantly lower rates of heart disease, cancer (especially colon cancer), and diabetes. What wonders to perform! But how much dietary fiber do we need?

Ways to Increase Fiber

The American Diet includes only 5 to 20 grams of dietary fiber per day. Recommendations range from 25 to 40 grams. The new required standard food labeling law lists 25 grams. Aim toward 40 grams. Emphasizing one kind of fiber, such as the insoluble fibers, by sprinkling wheat bran into everything or taking high-fiber food supplements is inadequate. The best way to get the full range of dietary fibers is to make 45% to 65% of your calorie intake* unrefined carbohydrates. Include a variety of fresh vegetables,

---

* See Calorie Chart, p. 98.
* Example: 45% to 65% of 1800 Calories = 810 to 1170 calories
  (.45 x 1800 = 810, .65 x 1800 = 1170)

fruits, whole grains, beans and peas, and nuts and seeds. The following chart gives the approximate dietary fiber in these foods. To ensure that our bodies get the benefits of dietary fiber variety, we also need to drink plenty of water, spread fiber foods throughout all the meals of the day, and eat lots of raw foods. Cooking vegetables does not decrease the fiber, but stir-frying and steaming seem to be the best preparation methods. To avoid the problems of gas or diarrhea, ease into a high-fiber diet. It takes time for the digestive system to become accustomed to an increase in fiber. You may read that high fiber can prevent some important minerals from being absorbed by the body. Don't worry about this. It can happen initially as you adjust, but in the long run, a wide variety of plant foods and a level of 30 to 40 grams of dietary fiber should not create this problem. Don't worry about adjustments in amounts for different ages. Amounts for children will automatically be adjusted by the amount of food they eat.

If you have any chronic health condition such as colon problems or diabetes, it is important to consult your physician about the best way to gradually add dietary fiber to your diet.

Happy fibrous eating!

Dietary Fiber in Foods

Amounts listed supply about 4 grams of dietary fiber each.*

Whole grains, flours, breads, cereals	Amount
barley, uncooked	1¼ cup
bran, oat, dry	3 tablespoons
bran, wheat, dry	¼ cup
bulgur wheat (Ala)	½ cup dry
cornmeal, stoneground	¼ cup
corn tortillas	10
Grape Nuts	¼ cup
millet cereal, cooked	1 cup
Nutri-Grain, Kellogg's (Almond Raisin)	1 cup
popped corn	2½ cups
rice, brown	1½ cup
rice, white	5 cups
rolled oats, uncooked	½ cup
Roman Meal, uncooked	⅓ cup
rye bread	2½ slices
rye crackers, wafers	5
rye flour, dark	¼ cup
shredded wheat	2 large biscuits
shredded wheat, spoon size	1 cup
Wheatena, cooked	1¼ cup
Wheaties	2 cups
whole-wheat bread	2½ slices
whole-wheat flour	2 cups
Total (General Mills)	2 cups

Legumes (dry beans, peas, cooked)	
black beans	¼ cup
black-eyed peas	¼ cup
broad beans	1 cup
garbanzos (chickpeas)	⅓ cup
kidney beans	1⅛ cup
lentils	⅓ cup
lima beans	1½ cup
pinto beans	⅔ cup
split peas	⅓ cup
soybeans	1½ cup
white beans	½ cup

---

* No standard laboratory measurement of dietary fiber has been established. Different tables give slightly varying measures in different foods. Dietary fiber data is also given for all recipes in the *Eating Better Cookbooks* (see p. 383 for information).

Fruits, uncooked

apple with skin	1 (4 oz.)
applesauce (cooked)	1¼ cup
avocado, 10 oz.	1
bananas, medium	2
blackberries	½ cup
blueberries	4 cups
cherries, sweet	44
cranberries	3 cups
dates	1 cup
figs, dried, small	5
grapefruit	2 halves
orange, small-medium	2
pears, small with skin	2
plums, small	5
pineapple	2½ cups
prunes, dried	3
raisins	6 tablespoons
raspberries	⅔ cup
strawberries	1 cup
tangerines, medium	2

Vegetables, uncooked

bean sprouts	1¼ cup
cabbage	2 cups
carrot, large	1
cauliflower	2 cups
celery stalks (4 oz.)	3
cucumber, 10-inch (8 oz.)	2½ cups
lettuce	4-5 cups
radishes	1⅓ cup
spinach	4-5 leaves

Vegetables, cooked

artichoke, medium	1
asparagus	1 cup
beans, green snap	1 cup
beets	1 cup
broccoli	1 cup
brussels sprouts	½ cup
cabbage	1½ cup
carrots	1 cup
collards	1 cup
corn	½ cup
cauliflower	2 cups
eggplant	2 cups
kale	1 cup
onions	1¼ cup
parsnips	½ cup

Vegetables, cooked cont.

peas, green	½ cup
potatoes	1 cup
baked, small-medium	1
rutabagas	1¼ cup
spinach	1 cup
squash, summer	1 cup
squash, winter	1⅛ cup
sweet potato, large (yam, U.S. variety)	1
tomatoes	1 cup
turnips	1 cup
zucchini	1 cup

Nuts and seeds

almonds, slivered	1½ cups
whole	40
cashews	1⅛ cup
coconut	¾ cup
peanuts with skins	1¼ cup
pecans	16
sesame seeds, whole	½ cup
sunflower seeds	¾ cup
walnuts	2¼ tablespoons

Calorie Chart*

Use this chart to learn what foods are low-, moderate-, and high-calorie. "Accounting for every calorie" is not essential to the *Eating Better Lifestyle*. The amounts listed are approximate ranges only.

Count 0 calories for average serving size

celery
cucumber
lettuce
mushrooms
onions
radishes
raw spinach
alfalfa sprouts
bean sprouts, raw
mustard
soy sauce
vinegar
lemon juice
lime juice
herb or black tea
decaffeinated coffee

Count 50 calories

Fruits:
1/2 cup:
grapes
blackberries
blueberries
loganberries
pineapple
cherries
unsweetened applesauce
unsweetened canned fruits
1 cup:
strawberries
raspberries
melons

Count 50 calories

Pieces:
1/2 grapefruit
1 peach
1 fig
1 orange
1 tangelo
1 tangerine
1 quince
1 kiwi fruit
2-3 dates
2-3 plums
3-4 apricots

Vegetables:
1/2 cup:
corn
peas
canned tomatoes
winter squash
ripe olives
pasta or tomato sauce
1 cup:
cabbage (raw)
dark leafy greens (cooked)
spinach, collards, kale,
turnip, mustard
bean sprouts (cooked)
okra
beets
broccoli
brussels sprouts
cauliflower (cooked)
carrots
rutabaga
eggplant

---

* For more specific calorie counts use the *Eating Better Cookbooks* (see p. 383 for information).

50 calories, Vegetables cont.

2 cups:
cauliflower (raw)
beet greens (cooked)
cabbage (cooked)
zucchini
vegetable salads, most

Pieces:
1 artichoke
1 large carrot
1 large tomato
8-12 asparagus spears

Breads, crackers, cereals:
1 cup puffed cereals
1 cup plain popcorn
6-inch corn tortilla
2 brown rice cakes
2 triple Rykrisp

Nuts and seeds:
1 tablespoon chopped (most)
2–3 tablespoons coconut

Dairy products:
2 tablespoons Parmesan
cheese
1 tablespoon cream cheese
1½ tablespoons sour cream
½ cup nonfat plain yogurt
1 medium egg

Sweets and spreads:
1 tablespoon honey or fructose
1 tablespoon jam
1 tablespoon maple syrup
1 tablespoon sorghum
3 tablespoons catsup

Count 100 calories

Fruits:
1 nectarine
1 small mango
1 small papaya
1 pear
1 small persimmon
1 pomegranate
1 small banana
¼ avocado
fruit salads, most

Count 100 calories

Fruits, dried:
¼ cup raisins
¼ cup dried apricots
5 prunes, dried
1 slice dried pineapple

Fruit juices:
¾ to 1 cup

Vegetables:
5 oz. (small) Irish potato
⅓ cup sweet potato
⅓ cup yam (U.S. variety)
7-inch ear corn

Breads, cereals:
½ cup brown rice (cooked)
½ cup bulgur (cooked)
½ cup pasta (cooked)
macaroni, noodles, spaghetti
1 oz. serving cold or hot cereals (¼
to 1 cup—check cereal box)
1 slice (1.5 oz.) whole-grain bread
1 whole-wheat tortilla
1 whole-wheat pita bread
½ whole-wheat English muffin
1 whole-grain dinner roll
4 (1 oz.) Akmak whole-wheat
crackers
1 cookie
gelatin dessert

Dairy products:
¼ cup (1 oz.) cheddar cheese
⅓ cup ricotta cheese

½ cup:
low-fat cottage cheese
whole milk
low-fat plain yogurt
low-fat vanilla yogurt
nonfat fruit yogurt
tofu

¾ cup (6 oz.):
buttermilk
low-fat milk
1 large or extra-large egg

Meats:
⅓ cup tuna

100 calories, Meats cont.

4-oz. serving lean fish:
bass
haddock
halibut
ocean perch
pollock
snapper
cod
flounder

3-oz. fish:
bluefish
carp
catfish
swordfish

Fats:
1 tablespoon:
butter
vegetable oil
mayonnaise
peanut butter

Count 150 calories
1 whole-grain muffin

Count 200 calories

Meat, fish, poultry:
4-oz. serving fatty fish:
herring
mackerel
salmon
shad
whitefish

3.5-oz. or ³/₄ cup:
chicken
turkey
¹/₂ cup ground turkey

4-oz. serving red meats:
beef chuck
flank steak
round steak
lean ground beef
leg of lamb
meat loaf

Nuts and seeds:
¹/₄ cup chopped

Count 200 calories

Sweets:
¹/₄ cup maple syrup

Dry wine:
1 cup

Count 200 to 400 calories

(check amounts of individual recipes)
casseroles, most
sandwiches, most
soups, most
cakes and desserts, most

Count 300 calories

Meats, red—4-oz. serving:
rump roast
sirloin steak
regular ground beef
lamb, shoulder, chops

Breads:
4 whole-grain pancakes
average serving waffles

Sweet wine:
1 cup

Count 400 calories

meats, red—4-oz. serving:
rib roast
club steak
porterhouse steak
T-bone steak
1 piece pie (¹/₈ pie)

Count over 400 calories (highest)

average serving:
quiches
bean burritos
tostada, meatless or not
pizza
beef or turkey burgers
some cheesy and/or meaty
 casseroles
1 piece double-crust pie (¹/₈ pie)

20

Plenty of Protein!

*D*epending on weight, our bodies need 40 to 60 grams of protein daily. Protein, the primary building material for the body, helps in forming the hormones and enzymes, in maintaining water balance and acid/base balance in the body, in forming mother's milk, and in clotting of blood. Surely it is one of our Lord's nutrient marvels!

Fortunately, protein deficiency is uncommon in the United States. In fact, the American Diet contains twice as much protein as needed. The concern that meat or dairy products are essential for adequate protein intake is unfounded. Getting plenty of protein into meals through a variety of whole foods in good balance is very easy—much easier than getting enough dietary fiber in and getting excessive fat out! How do we do it?

The protein that our bodies need consists of a combination of 22 amino acids. They are called "the building blocks" of the protein molecule. Eight of these are called essential amino acids because they cannot be manufactured in the body. They are tryptophan, leucine, isoleucine, lysine, valine, threonine, methionine, and cystine. A ninth, histidine, is essential for young children and possibly for adults. Practically every food has some of the essential amino acids—even fruits, although they have the least. Vegetables contain a little more, and grains, beans, nuts, and seeds are even higher. All of these unrefined carbohydrates are called incomplete proteins because none of them adequately supplies all eight essential amino acids. In contrast, meat, fish, poultry, eggs, and dairy products do contain all eight and are therefore called complete proteins.

It has been thought that all eight essential amino acids must be eaten at the same meal to get the full benefit of them all. That's why we have come to understand that we need animal foods for protein. Yet all of the essential amino acids are supplied in our carbohydrate foods when we eat them in a good variety. Some combinations of incomplete protein will make complete protein dishes. For example, grains are low in lysine but beans are not. When the two are combined, complete protein is formed. In addition, when complete protein foods such as milk, eggs, or cheese are combined with incomplete protein foods such as grains, the protein value of the grains is increased. Combinations of complex carbohydrates that make complete protein are:

> *grains and beans*—such as chili and cornbread, peanut butter and bread, lentils and rice, baked beans and brown bread
>
> *grains and dark leafy greens*—such as rice pilaf and spinach salad
>
> *grains and dairy products*—such as macaroni and cheese, toasted cheese sandwich, muffins or pancakes made with milk and eggs

beans and sesame or sunflower seeds—such as garbanzo spread or falafel, kidney beans and sunflower seeds in a salad

These are called complementary protein combinations. The need for these combinations in one meal has probably been overrated. Actually, including these foods regularly at any time in our meals in any combination is sufficient to supply adequate protein. The key is variety. In countries where variety is unavailable, protein deficiencies can occur. Communities that rely on corn, for example, can be deficient in lysine. A high-lysine corn has been developed to work toward meeting such needs as this. We would do well to think seriously about those who are in much greater need than ourselves. Then we will begin to be thankful for the incredible variety that is ours!

21

The Slippery Subject of Fats!

———— ♥ ————

So there was food every day for Elijah and for the woman and her family. For the jar of flour was not used up and the jug of oil did not run dry, in keeping with the word of the LORD spoken by Elijah.

1 Kings 17:15,16

———— ♥ ————

*H*ave you ever tried to explain something simply and clearly and then realized that your explanations raised more questions than answers? So it is with the subject of fats! If ever new products have been promoted on fear, this is it. In the 1980s, along with salt, cholesterol became practically synonymous with sin. In the 1990s our focus has been turned to fat, low-fat, and fat-free! Advertising provides simple and often wrong solutions.

Nutritional research, however, is quite a different matter. There are more questions than answers. The result is that you and I see contradiction and controversy that leaves us confused. What are we going to do? First, let's find out what fat is good for, what kinds of fats there are, and then which ones are our best choices.

We've put some foods that involve the fat issue into other chapters—meats, eggs, and dairy products. Therefore, we won't discuss these foods in much detail in this chapter, but will focus on the almost exclusively concentrated fats—vegetable oils and butter.

We Need Some Fat!

First of all, fat in itself is not bad. Our bodies need fat to transport the fat-soluble vitamins (A, D, E, and K), to convert carotene from plant foods to vitamin A, to protect vital organs, to regulate temperature, to provide a concentrated source of energy, to provide the essential fatty acids (linoleic and linolenic acid), to satiate hunger, and to add wonderful flavor to many dishes.

Even cholesterol is not bad. Cholesterol is a necessary part of all body cells, especially nerve, brain, blood, and liver cells. It assists in nutrient and waste transport in and out of the cells, assists in the forming of bile and vital hormones, and lubricates the skin. Our bodies use much more cholesterol than our food provides, and manufacture what needed cholesterol is not consumed in food. We do not want to cast fat aside, but to regulate it.

What Kinds of Fat Are There?

Just as with dietary fiber, all fats are not in the same form. The four basic known forms of fat are polyunsaturated, saturated, monounsaturated, and cholesterol. All vegetable oils contain a combination of the first three forms but no cholesterol. Some vegetable oils are high in polyunsaturates, such as safflower oil (77%), flaxseed oil (73%), sunflower oil (69%), corn oil (62%), and soybean oil (61%). Some are more highly saturated such as cottonseed oil

(26%), palm oil (51%), palm kernel oil (86%), and coconut oil (92%). These highly saturated oils are used in prepackaged processed foods. They have also been traditionally used for frying in restaurants and fast-food outlets, although there is a growing trend to replace them with polyunsaturated fats. Monounsaturated oils contain a higher percentage of monounsaturated fat—olive oil (77%), canola oil (62%), and peanut oil (48%). The fat of avocados is also primarily monounsaturated.

All animal fats contain a combination of saturated, polyunsaturated, and monounsaturated fats, plus cholesterol. Among animal foods, fish are lowest in saturated fat and cholesterol, and contain valuable polyunsaturated omega-3 fatty acids.

How Fat Can Affect Weight Control

The confusion and controversy surrounding these forms of fat involves their various effects on health in special regard to cancers, heart disease, and weight control. The least confusing issue is the effect of fats on weight control. All fats, no matter what form, contain nine calories per gram—twice as many calories as a gram of protein or carbohydrate. A high-fat diet, very simply, adds too many calories too easily for most people, especially in combination with a refined carbohydrate diet that contains inadequate dietary fibers. Limiting overall intake of fat of all kinds is a very effective way to control calorie levels.

Other Problems with Fats and Oils

Many research studies have shown a correlation between heart disease and fats. The most well-established link to date is that diets that are higher in saturated fats do raise blood cholesterol levels—a leading contributor to heart-disease risk. This is the reason that we have been cautioned to reduce meats and dairy products and encouraged to use more vegetable oils, because they are much higher in polyunsaturated fat. Other research shows that polyunsaturates reduce blood cholesterol. Yet, other studies indicate that too much polyunsaturated oil may lead to certain forms of cancer. One reason for this is the high susceptibility of polyunsaturated vegetable oils to rancidity. Rancid oils in the body are carcinogenic. Refinement of oils extracts the vitamin E, which acts as a natural preservative. Heating oils in cooking compounds the risk of rancidity. It also converts some of the *cis* form of polyunsaturated oil to the *trans* form (now implicated in both heart disease and cancers). Saturated and monounsaturated fats are less susceptible to this conversion. It is actually better for deep-fat-fried foods (if you are going to eat them) to be fried in the more stable saturated fats such as coconut or palm oil.

What About Hydrogenated Vegetable Fat, Margarine, and Butter?

Added to the extraction of nutrients in oil processing is the hydrogenation of fat. Hydrogenation adds an extra hydrogen molecule to give oils a longer shelf life. Oils lightly hydrogenated will be thicker, yet still liquid at room temperature. Heavily hydrogenated oils will be solid at room temperature. All vegetable shortenings and margarines are hydrogenated. Hydrogenation increases the saturation of fats. Vegetable shortenings are often made from more highly saturated fats to begin with, such as Crisco which is made from hydrogenated soybean and palm oil (51% saturated). Hydrogenation also changes the natural *cis* form of fatty acids into *trans* fatty acids. Some nutritionists maintain that the body cannot utilize the *trans* form of fatty acids. According to Warren N. Levin, M.D., member of the International Academy of Preventive Medicine, "These trans-fatty acids do not fit into the body machinery and tend to 'gum up the works.'"[1] Therefore, Dr. Levin recommends butter over margarine, although butter is a saturated fat. Carlton Fredericks, Ph.D., also wrote in regard to margarine in "Hotline to Health," *Prevention*

(December 1980, p. 39), "A recent report in the *Journal of Nutrition* (October 1979, pp. 1759-65) warns that excessive intake of trans fats tends to aggravate existing deficiencies in essential fatty acids." We are inclined to agree with these findings on the basis that man's chemical alterations of real foods repeatedly have been found wanting in their effects upon human health. There may be quite a bit we don't know concerning the effects of trans fatty acids on human health that we will wish later that we did know. For these reasons we recommend using real butter or vegetable oil in baking, and *Butter Spread* (recipe, p. 371) or real butter for spread. *Butter Spread* is a combination of equal parts butter and canola or safflower oil, reducing the portion of saturated fat and increasing the portion of valuable essential fatty acids.

In the meantime, as we have been faced with this fat dilemma, modern research is turning up exciting new information about olive oil, canola oil, flaxseed oil, and fish.

Olive Oil

New studies indicate that olive oil, a monounsaturated fat, is also effective in lowering blood cholesterol levels without having the dangers in relationship to cancers that polyunsaturated fats do. In addition, olive oil assists bowel regularity, and "is easily digested, imparting a soothing and healing influence to the digestive tract. This healing and cleansing effect is due to the high content of potassium and also sodium and calcium."[2] Olive oil is the primary vegetable oil used regularly in Mediterranean countries. People in this area do not suffer the high incidence of heart disease that we do in America. We are quite excited about these findings. Olive oil has been spoken of well in the Bible: "Observe the commands of the LORD your God, walking in his ways and revering him. For the LORD your God is bringing you into a good land—a land with streams and pools of water, with springs flowing in the valleys and hills; a land with wheat and barley, vines and fig trees, pomegranates, olive oil and honey" (Deuteronomy 8:6-8), and "every one of you will eat from his own vine and fig tree and drink water from his own cistern, until I come and take you to a land like your own, a land of grain and new wine, a land of bread and vineyards, a land of olive trees and honey. Choose life and not death!" (2 Kings 18:31,32).

Reducing our use of polyunsaturated vegetable oils is a wise idea. Replace some of it with olive oil. Olive oil can even be used in most baking without its flavor coming through—even more strong-flavored extra virgin olive oil. Try Emilie's gourmet *Olive Oil Dressing* (p. 372), a recipe from her father, who was a famous Viennese chef.

Canola Oil

Of our commonly used oils, canola oil has a most advantageous balance of the three types of fat: 62% monounsaturated, 32% polyunsaturated, and a low 6% saturated. Both essential fatty acids are provided in ample amounts— 22% linoleic, and 10% linolenic. It is a good all-purpose oil, mild in flavor, and reasonable in cost. While we do prefer olive oil for baking and sautéeing when the flavor is compatible, we occasionally use canola oil, especially for *Butter Spread* (p. 371). The main reason to minimize use of canola oil over direct heat and to use olive oil in baking when compatible with flavor is that canola oil is higher in polyunsaturated fat that more easily breaks down into harmful compounds when subjected to high heat (see p. 107).

Flaxseed Oil

Flaxseed oil has been used for centuries in Europe. It is costly and highly perishable. Of all the oils, it contains the highest portion of the harder-to-get essential fatty acid, linolenic. In fact, flaxseed oils is 57% linolenic acid plus 18% linoleic acid. Linolenic acid is an omega-3 fatty acid, valuable for controlling cholesterol and triglycerides.

Flaxseed oil may be obtained from the refrigerator case in a health-food store in small (about 8 oz.) bottles. We use small amounts in our tossed salads. We also use freshly ground flax seeds in shakes, on top of hot cereal, in cottage cheese, and over fresh fruit. Flax seeds are less perishable than the oil and much less expensive. We store both oil and seeds in the freezer. An inexpensive coffee bean grinder works perfectly for grinding small amounts of flax seed. For more information on olive, canola, and flaxseed oils and their uses, see *Eating Better Breakfasts* and *Eating Better Main Dishes* (p. 384).

Selection and Care of Quality Oils

We recommend using the highest quality of oil that your budget will allow. Choose organic extra virgin olive oil, pure expeller pressed canola oil, and expeller pressed safflower oil. We suggest *Arrowhead Mills, Omega Nutrition*, or *Spectrum Naturals* brands. These may be purchased at health food stores. Oils of this quality are admittedly expensive, but this can be a blessing in disguise, as this should prevent most of us from using too much. Fats and oils is the most seriously misunderstood food issue in America. Get a copy of *The Facts About Fats* by John Finnegan—"must" reading (see Recommended Reading, p. 380).

Keep all oil, except olive oil, in the refrigerator, and flaxseed oil which is best kept in the freezer.

Fat Fish Story

The new discovery in fish is EPA and DHA (called omega-3 fatty acids), two polyunsaturated fatty acids that lower blood cholesterol and triglycerides. Fatty fish are highest in EPA and DHA, and include mackerel, salmon, blue fish, sardines, mullet, rainbow trout, lake trout, herring, tuna, sable fish, shad, butterfish, and pompano. No one knows yet how much fish will accomplish these health effects, but one suggestion is two to four fish meals a week in contrast to the average American's one fish meal a week. Fish is easily digested and very high in protein. Weston A. Price, D.D.S., who toured the world to extensively study the health condition of over 100 tribal groups in the 1940s, reported in his book *Nutrition and Physical Degeneration* that the strongest, most energetic people groups were those who had access to seafoods. The Eskimos who have lived on a very high fat whale meat diet have not suffered from heart disease. The Japanese whose diets are high in seafoods have also enjoyed a low incidence of heart trouble.

Eating even one more fish meal a week than we now eat will count for better health. See page 116 for some cautions on the kinds of fish to choose.

Flaxseed oil and flax seeds, as already mentioned, also provide the omega-3 fatty acid, linolenic acid. The value of flaxseed, fish oils, and monunsaturated oils to the control of blood cholesterol are testimony that, although some types of fat apparently raise cholesterol levels, other types control or lower cholesterol levels. Thus, it is a serious mistake to dismiss all fat from the diet. Quality fats, rather, make a valuable contribution, perhaps even of more importance than limiting fat intake to 30% or less of calories.

Cholesterol-Lowering Foods

Some interesting studies reveal that certain foods can lower blood cholesterol levels. For example, a group of men was given 18 tablespoons of oat bran a day for ten days. Their blood cholesterol drop averaged 18%.[3] Most people would not consume on a regular daily diet so much of any one food. We do not yet know how much of any one food or a combination of foods in a normal diet might assist in regulating cholesterol levels. Foods that may contribute to normal blood cholesterol levels, however, include garlic, onions, avocados, eggplant, seeds, cabbage, soybeans, peanuts, oats, oat bran, beans, yams, and barley. Both dietary fibers and other properties, including vitamins and minerals, in these foods are of value. There may be other whole foods, as well, that we may discover that contribute to the body's ability to handle fats properly. For example, a recent study revealed that those who included five hand-fuls of nuts in their weekly diet, suffer fewer heart attacks than those who don't. Nuts are another of God's whole-food packages combining vitamin E, dietary fiber and other vitamins and minerals along with high-quality fat. All these foods may work together synergistically (p. 86) for our health.

A Fat Menu to
Keep You from Slipping

Include more fish, especially the fatty kind.
Use a little flaxseed and olive oil,
and leave some of those polys* behind!
Let the hydroges* on the shelf remain—
that means the shortening,
the "partiallys,"*
and the mar-gar-ine.
Use nuts and seeds often,
but fresh and few;
chew them well for great taste,
crunch, and nutrients, too!
Also eating fresh ground flax seed
would be a good thing to do!
And opt for real butter or Butter Spread,*
but just a tad
Keep fats below 30% of cals,*
and you'll be glad!
Or 10 to 20% if you want to
shed a pound or two.
When it comes to fat, use a wise head,
Don't give them all up,
Use good quality instead!

—Sue Gregg

---

* polyunsaturated fats, hydrogenated fats, partially hydrogenated fats, calories. Keep concentrated vegetable and butter fats to 1 to 2 tablespoons per day. *Butter Spread* recipe, p. 371.

22

Is Meat a Menace to Your Health?

———— ♥ ————

Do not join those who drink too much wine or gorge
themselves on meat, for drunkards and gluttons become
poor, and drowsiness clothes them in rags.

Proverbs 23:20,21

———— ♥ ————

*A*mericans consume 30% of the world's animal protein, yet we are only 7% of the world's population.
Worldwide, the more affluent a society becomes and the
more influenced by Western civilization, the more meat-
centered it becomes. The meat-centered diet reflects the
belief that we must have it to meet our protein needs. In
fact, many homemakers don't know how to plan a menu
without it. In the meantime, vegetarians are enjoying less
incidence of diabetes, high blood pressure, osteoporosis,
high estrogen levels and gallstones in women, high blood
cholesterol levels, heart disease, and hormone-related cancer in men (such as prostate).

The quality of our meat is not what it once was a short 50 years ago. Beef used to be a lean 5% to 10% fat when cattle were range-fed on grasses and matured over two to three years. Today high-energy feeds and 18 months of fast growth marbleizes the beef with over 30% saturated fat. Meat production has become a huge economic enterprise requiring over 2700 drugs including antibiotics, hormones, tranquilizers, and pesticides. More drugs are used by cattlemen than by medical doctors. Chemical residues inevitably remain in the meat and cannot be cooked out.

Among the food groups, animal products are the most highly susceptible to bacterial contamination. In fact salmonella contamination is so high that testing for it has not been considered worth the time. In 1987 the USDA reported that "Nearly four out of every ten chickens sold to consumers are contaminated by salmonella. . . ."[1] Millions suffer yearly from these contaminated meats. For example, between 1971 and 1983 there were over 15 million estimated associations of salmonella illness with meat and poultry.[2] Scientists estimate that about 30% of the 69 million to 275 million cases of diarrhea that occur each year result from food contamination.[3] Although salmonella can be destroyed through proper cooking, bacteria can be carried from hands contaminated with infected raw meat to other foods. The most frequent victims are the elderly, the sick, the unborn, and infants.

Pigs and shellfish have always been scavengers by nature. That means that they act like living garbage cans. High quality feed notwithstanding, pigs cannot be divorced from their scavenger nature. They will eat their own feces even in the most carefully controlled situations.

The danger of pork, improperly cooked, has been understood as trichinosis, caused by a parasite that can enter the body through pork that has been eaten. *The Albany Democrat-Herald* (Saturday, October 11, 1980) carried an article entitled, "Trichinosis now affects only about 2% of U.S. population, Center for Disease Control reports." Two percent of the American population is approximately 4½ million people. "Most don't even know they are infected and the cases never are reported."

Industrial wastes poured into lakes, rivers, and oceans are slowly contaminating our fish supply as well. Freshwater fish from inland lakes and rivers are the most contaminated, especially with PCB's. Swordfish and carp contain the highest mercury levels. Deep-ocean fish and smaller fish are less likely to be contaminated. Pregnant women especially should avoid high levels of both PCB's and mercury. Fresh fish can also be sprayed with chemicals to help preserve freshness before it is sold.

Historically, people have eaten very small amounts of meat compared to complex carbohydrates. Even at the turn of the century, Americans ate less than half the meat eaten today although their protein intake was about the same. Animal foods are more difficult to digest than plant foods. Fish is the easiest meat to digest, followed by poultry.

———— ♥ ————

Our recipes and menus in Part 7 give you ideas for both meatless meals and meals with small amounts of meat. We suggest a goal of serving three meat meals a week at most. Replace red meats with fish and poultry. You might serve chicken one evening, turkey or lamb another evening, fish a third evening. Fish might be served more frequently, however. Replace regular ground beef with ground turkey. It is lower in calories and fat, and poultry is easier for the body to digest. Ground turkey contains turkey skin, however, so it is higher in fat than turkey dark meat and light meat. Aim for serving smaller amounts of meat in stir-fry dishes and casseroles.

Try to purchase meats that have been grown without drugs. These may be labeled "organically grown." Call your local health-food store, a local food co-op, and check resources (pp. 304-06). Do not purchase beef or chicken livers unless grown without drugs. The liver is a dumping ground for toxic residues. Use only fresh or frozen meats. Avoid processed meats with preservatives such as nitrites or nitrates, or with refined sugars added.

When you prepare meats, wash your hands thoroughly before handling other food, dishes, utensils, or cleaning supplies. Cut meats on a hard plastic cutting board that you can wash in the dishwasher. Use a different board for cutting other foods. Thaw all your meats in the refrigerator or the microwave, preferably in the refrigerator (see pp. 191-92). Don't leave any meats, cooked or raw, standing at room temperature over two hours. Bacteria multiply rapidly between 40° F. and 140° F. Cook poultry and meats thoroughly without interrupting the process.

To reduce fat content, remove skin from chicken and turkey. Trim all the visible fat from meats. Bake, broil, or fry in nonstick pans and drain off all excess fat. Charcoal broiling produces high amounts of benzoprene residue, a carcinogen related to leukemia and stomach cancer.[4]

It is a fact that, on any given day, 80% of Americans see very little, if any, fresh produce on their plates. The American Diet chart (p. 38) illustrates this. Gary Null in *The New Vegetarian* reminds us that "meat eaters' diets are likely to be much more restricted than vegetarians' diets. . . . When meat is the center of the meal, contributions from other food groups (grains, legumes, fruits, and vegetables) are often kept to minimum servings."[5] By reducing our dependency on meats as the focus of our menu planning, we are free to enjoy a greater variety of God's cornucopia of whole foods.

Let me state it clearly. We have drastically reduced the amount of meat we eat and probably eat red meat about one or two times a year. Most of our meals are vegetarian meals. But we are not vegetarians. Vegetarianism has its limitations, too, though it's nutritionally not so severe as the American Diet. But there is a spiritual base to much of the current practice of vegetarianism that is a "must" for

Christians to understand (see chapter 38). This is especially true as the agendas of strict vegetarians, environmentalists, and animal right groups become more militant. If we are going to be meat eaters, we should have a biblical basis for it and know how to give an account of ourselves to the growing number of people who are of a different persuasion.

In addition, strict vegetarianism may not be the healthiest diet. Dr. Weston A. Price states in *Nutrition and Physical Degeneration:* "As yet I have not found a single group... which was building and maintaining excellent bodies by living entirely on plant foods. I have found in many parts of the world most devout representatives of modern ethical systems advocating the restriction of foods to the vegetable products. In every instance where the groups involved had been long under this teaching, I found evidence of degeneration in the form of dental caries, and in the new generation in the form of abnormal dental arches to an extent much higher than in the... groups who were not under this influence."[6]

23

Eggs—
Ample of Controversy!

———— ♥ ————

As an inexpensive source of good nutrition, there is
nothing more glorious than the egg.

Edward Ahrens

———— ♥ ————

The controversy and confusion over eggs focuses on the high cholesterol content of egg yolks. Media advertising, news articles, magazines, nutrition books, cookbooks, doctors, and nutritionists would have us believe that food cholesterol raises blood cholesterol. Yet there is no adequate research to substantiate this claim. Researchers are not agreed at all on this issue. The classic study that relates egg yolk cholesterol to blood cholesterol was conducted in 1913 by Nikolai Anichkov, a Russian pathologist, on rabbits. He fed rabbits the equivalent to human consumption of 60 eggs per day. The rabbits developed cholesterol deposits on their arteries. But rabbits are total vegetarians and do not eat eggs. "There is nothing in their metabolism to handle eggs."[1]

No human study shows a clear relationship between food cholesterol content and blood cholesterol, whereas research does indicate a clearer relationship to total fat consumption, especially to saturated fat. Yet eggs are lower in saturated fat than both meat and poultry, about the same as low-fat yogurt, and contain one-third of the amount that is in ¼ cup (1 oz.) of cheddar cheese.

Advertising and popular news articles repeatedly reinforce the notion that food cholesterol raises blood cholesterol levels. "No cholesterol" labels are printed on vegetable oils and advertised everywhere. The message is effectively communicated: "Cholesterol in foods must be bad!"

Time magazine, March 26, 1984, reported the most extensive research project ever conducted on cholesterol in medical history. This project has been declared "a turning point in cholesterol-heart-disease research,"[2] because it clearly demonstrated that high blood cholesterol contributes to heart disease and cardiac deaths. Ten years and $150 million were spent on 3806 men, ages 35 to 59 with cholesterol levels of 265 mg. A cholesterol-lowering drug was used in the study. Those receiving the drug experienced an 8.5% drop in cholesterol, 19% fewer heart attacks, and 24% fewer cardiac deaths. Yet nothing was changed in their diets. The study had nothing to do with cholesterol content of any foods.

The editors of *Time* magazine placed a "sad-face" picture on the front cover of its March 26, 1984, issue using two fried eggs for eyes and a slice of bacon for the mouth, with an overcaption of "Cholesterol . . . And Now the Bad News." On page 56 the article was entitled "Hold the Eggs and Butter." The message conveyed to the reader was that "eggs and butter contribute to heart disease." Yet the research project reviewed by *Time* had nothing to do with the effects of food on cholesterol! This kind of media influence confuses important nutritional issues for the American public.

Of this research project Edward Ahrens, researcher at Rockefeller University, said, "Since this was basically a drug study we can conclude nothing about diet; such extrapolation is unwarranted, unscientific and wishful thinking."[3]

Only 20% to 30% of our cholesterol comes from food. Our bodies manufacture the rest. There are many other influences on blood cholesterol levels besides total fat intake, such as exercise, stress, inherited genes, prepackaged foods high in fats and refined carbohydrates, lack of dietary fiber, and inadequate vitamins and minerals. Rather than focus on egg yolks as a dietary disaster, we should develop a balance of real whole foods.

Eggs are a real food. They can readily be used in baking and a couple of times a week for meals. Two breakfasts or an egg main dish will not raise the total fat intake to over 30% of calories. Eggs are our best protein source because their amino acid pattern most nearly matches that needed for human growth and health.[4] They are excellent sources of trace minerals, unsaturated fatty acids, iron, phosphorus, vitamin B-complex, A, E, K, and even some D. Most of these reside in the egg yolk! Yolks also are the highest food source of choline, a component of lecithin that assists in keeping cholesterol liquid in the bloodstream. There is some question as to whether the lecithin is effective in this way, however.

If you do not want to eat egg yolks or are allergic to eggs, be encouraged. There are easy alternatives! You can use two egg whites in place of a whole egg in almost any baking recipe. Unfortunately, that wastes the egg yolks. You might just as well use commercial *Egg Beaters* which are primarily egg whites. Other alternatives include *Ener-G Egg Replacer* (potato starch, tapioca base), available in health-food stores, arrowroot binder, and flaxseed binder (recipes in **Breakfasts**—see p. 384 for information). Flaxseed binder made from ground flax seeds is a nutritionally excellent replacement for eggs. Tofu also works in some recipes but can alter the texture. Use ¼ cup tofu in place of an egg. Soft tofu is best, blended thoroughly in a blender with other liquid ingredients. For alternatives to scrambled eggs and egg salad sandwich filling, try our *Tofu Scramble* (p. 342) and *Egg Real Fool! Sandwich* (p. 353).

Consider the value of fertile eggs. Fertile eggs come from hens, living with roosters, that are allowed to grow and peck on the ground. They receive no drugs as chickens raised in close quarters do. We don't really know what the nutritional difference between fertile eggs and sterile eggs is even though some people make claims for the nutritional superiority of fertile eggs. The clearest advantage is that fertile eggs are free of chemical residues. In general, fertile eggs also taste fresher but are also slightly more expensive. Many health-food stores carry them. People who raise their own chickens also often sell them.

Mankind has eaten eggs for centuries. Even Job ate eggs: ". . . is there flavor in the white of an egg? I refuse to touch it; such food makes me ill" (Job 6:6,7). Yet heart disease was not reported in scientific literature until 1896.[5] You decide. We still believe eggs are an economical blessing from God given to us to enjoy in moderation.

24

Are Dairy Products Deadly?

———— ♥ ————

The virgin . . . will call him Immanuel. He will eat curds and honey when he knows enough to reject the wrong and choose the right. . . . In that day, a man will keep alive a young cow and two goats. And because of the abundance of the milk they give, he will have curds to eat. All who remain in the land will eat curds and honey.
Isaiah 7:14,15,21,22

———— ♥ ————

*D*airy products can be an excellent, easily utilized form of protein, complementing vegetarian dishes. They are rich sources of calcium, vitamins A, D, E, K, and the B-vitamins, especially riboflavin. Some peoples with limited food variety have thrived on milk products and lived long, vigorous lives. Yet millions of Americans have difficulty with dairy products. What are the reasons and what are our options?

Health Problems

Milk is the number-one allergen in the United States. Many persons are also lactose (milk sugar) intolerant, especially those whose ancestral background did not include dairy products. Their bodies do not produce enough of the enzyme lactase to properly digest the lactose in milk products. The enzyme seems to decrease toward adulthood in many people.

Some nutritionists believe that milk is only for babies and remind us that no animal drinks milk past the weaning stage. Certainly most of us do well to reduce the amount of dairy products we use to cut fat and to make more room for fresh vegetables, fruits, grains, beans, nuts, and seeds in our diets. For some persons dairy products may cause mucous formation that contributes to congestion, poor digestion, colds, infections, and poor assimilation of nutrients.

Dairy products, as with meats, poultry, and fish, "now contain antibiotics, hormones, pesticides, radioactive isotopes, and other toxic materials—as well as, on occasion, disease-producing bacteria."[1]

Pasteurized Milk

The various forms of dairy products can also make a nutritional difference. Almost all milk is pasteurized. Pasteurization destroys about 38% of the vitamin B-complex, lowers vitamin B_{12} by 12%, destroys the vitamins A and C, reduces the availability of calcium by 10%, lowers protein digestibility by 4% and protein biological value by 17%, and destroys the digestive enzyme phosphatase.[2] Who knows what other unknown nutrient values are reduced or destroyed by pasteurization. Careful studies on animals all reveal better growth and health when raw milk is given. One such study performed on cats by Frances M. Pottenger, Jr., M.D. showed that cats fed pasteurized milk and cooked meat could not reproduce after the second generation. The cats on raw milk and raw meat did not develop this problem.[3] "Pasteurized milk was also tested against raw milk at the West of Scotland Agricultural College, by feeding them to comparable groups of calves. All the calves using the raw milk completed the test period satisfactorily. Those receiving only pasteurized milk became sick or died."[4]

The alternative to pasteurized milk is raw milk. Only raw certified milk is sufficiently safe raw milk, however. It is very unfortunate that it has limited availability, primarily to Southern California. The controversy over the safety of raw certified milk is very confusing. Raw certified milk is the only food product in the entire United States that undergoes testing for salmonella bacteria. There are millions of cases of salmonella illness from foods yearly, but Alta-Dena Dairy reported that in 13 years from 1971 through 1983 not one documented illness was ever traced to raw certified dairy products,[5] nor has there been a documented case at any time. In contrast, there have been many thousands of documented cases of illness traced directly to pasteurized milk in various parts of the country with some of the largest outbreaks in the 1980s. Pasteurization does not guarantee the safety of milk as effectively as the high cleanliness standards applied to raw certified milk.

Alta-Dena Dairy has the reputation of being the cleanest dairy in the United States. It was established by the Harold Steuve family with a vision for higher dairy standards to produce a safer milk supply. Alta-Dena Dairy has been a political target because its standards have been a threat to the dairy industry that uses pasteurization to compensate for poor standards of cleanliness. Alta-Dena has maintained the same high standards of cleanliness for its pasteurized milk as well. Alta-Dena raw certified dairy products are now sold under the brand name Steuve's Natural.

Media reports have seldom distinguished between raw milk that is not certified and raw certified milk when discussing the dangers of raw milk. There is risk in consuming any food product. Statistically both our meat and poultry

supply and pasteurized milk have proven to be less safe
than raw certified milk. We regret that many of our readers
cannot enjoy the freedom of choosing the benefits of raw
certified milk. In some areas of the country local brands of
raw milk are available.

Homogenized Milk

A discussion about raw certified milk is important even
if our readers cannot obtain it, because most pasteurized
milk is also homogenized. There may be serious problems
with homogenized milk as well. The fat molecules in homogenized milk have been altered to keep the fat from rising to
the top. This prolongs the shelf life of the milk. *The XO
Factor** by Kurt A. Oster, M.D., and Donald J. Ross, Ph.D.,
details and documents 40 years of research concerning the
enzyme xanthine oxidase, present in cow's milk. Their
research shows that a significant amount of xanthine oxidase gets into the bloodstream with the smaller fat molecules of homogenized milk and damages the arterial walls.
In turn, the body draws cholesterol, calcium, and other
protective agents from the bloodstream to repair the dam-
aged walls. Researchers admit openly that they do not
know the cause of initial damage to artery walls that trig-
gers the process of cholesterol deposits. "Scientists are not
yet certain why high levels of cholesterol lead to heart disease or what sets the insidious process in motion. The most
widely accepted explanation is the so-called injury theory,
propounded by Russell Ross at the University of Washington in Seattle. According to Ross, 'the disease begins with
damage to the thin layer of cells, or endothelium, that
forms the protective lining of the arteries.'"[6] Perhaps there
are several causes from our faulty diet. Could xanthine
oxidase be one of them?

**Homogenized!* by Nicolas Sampsidis, M.S., presents a shorter and easy-
to-read account of Oster's and Ross's work.

It is unfortunate that the scientific community has not yet seen fit to set aside vested interests and objectively investigate this theory. A historical lesson may remind us not to place total confidence upon orthodox views. In the nineteenth century Ignaz Semmelweis discovered that women died in childbirth because disease was carried in hospitals from person to person with doctors' unwashed hands. Semmelweis developed a method of hand washing that saved many lives. Yet his theory was not only rejected, he was also dismissed from his hospital position, and the antiseptic method of cleansing hands and instruments was not officially introduced until over 30 years later. It was not until 1960 that a book describing a method of washing the hands approximating the biblical method in Numbers 19 was written by the New York State Department of Health following a staph infection epidemic in 1958 caused by improperly washed hands.[7] While we wait for the scientific community to respond to the research regarding xanthine oxidase, we suggest caution in using homogenized milk as a dietary mainstay for our children.

Milk Choices

What are our options? Our first option is whole milk. Whole milk may provide more fat than many people desire. Yet when the fat is removed, so are most of the fat-soluble vitamins A, D, E, and K. The presence of fat is valuable to the assimilation of these nutrients. Although vitamins A and D are synthetically restored to skim or nonfat milk, we wonder how well this fortification matches the original nutrient value, or how well these are actually assimilated. Low-fat milk is a compromise between skim or nonfat and whole milk. What forms of whole, low-fat, or nonfat milk do we recommend?

Goat's milk is a wonderful choice because it is closer in composition to human milk than cow's milk. If you have access to it and it fits into your food budget, by all means take advantage of it. We have chosen to use Alta-Dena or

Steuve's Natural raw certified milk products because they are available to us. We make our own low-fat milk by blending equal amounts of raw certified whole milk and nonfat milk. We also use raw certified butter, buttermilk, cottage cheese, kefir, Jack cheese, and cheddar cheeses. Some of these latter raw certified products are available in many states throughout the U.S.A.

If raw certified milk is unavailable, we recommend nonfat or skim milk, or one of the alternative milk recipes in *Eating Better Breakfasts* (see p. 384). Skim milk may be fortified by blending in nonfat dry milk powder from the health-food store or instant nonfat dry milk from the supermarket. Add at least ⅓ cup per quart of nonfat milk, allowing it to refrigerate several hours to improve flavor. Nonfat dry milk can also be added freely to fortify baked goods. Use it as a replacement for half the sugar taken out of a recipe when honey is used. Keep in mind that nonfat milk will not provide original fat-soluble vitamins. Therefore, be certain to also include plenty of whole grains, and dark green and yellow vegetables in the menu.

If homogenized milk is used, xanthine oxidase can be inactivated by simmering at 195° F. for 10 to 15 seconds. This will alter the taste.

If you have a milk sugar (lactose) intolerance, inquire of your doctor, a nutritionist, or your local health-food store for new products that assist the body to digest it better. Digestive enzyme preparations, Lactaid or Lactase, are available at drugstores without prescription. Acidophilus milk or Lactaid are other options, though perhaps not the best (see *Eating Better Breakfasts* [see pp. 383-84 for ordering information]).

Cultured Milks

Cultured milks include yogurt, kefir, and buttermilk. When raw certified milk is not available, cultured milks are perhaps the best alternative available. They are easier to digest because part of the milk lactose has been converted to lactic acid. Even some persons allergic to sweet milk can tolerate some form of cultured milk. Yogurt and kefir contain live bacteria cultures that help the body to produce its own friendly bacteria in the colon to fight toxic bacteria and to produce its own B-vitamins. Not all yogurt is prepared with live bacteria. Any yogurt labeled with only gelatin added is not made with live bacteria. Yogurt with live bacteria will be labeled "viable cultures," "live bacteria," "lactobacillus acidophilus," or "acidophilus cultures." Also, we recommend yogurt not sweetened with refined sugars. Nonfat and low-fat yogurts are best unless pasteurized, nonhomogenized whole yogurt is available such as *Trader Joe's* brand (Southern California), or *Brown Cow* brand. As with milk, for the assimilation of fat-soluble nutrients we recommend this quality whole yogurt, especially for children.

Yogurt may also be made at home. Three yogurt recipes and a wonderful lesson in "The Art and Science of Yogurt Making" for children is available in *Eating Better Breakfasts* (see p. 384). No raw certified yogurt is commercially available.

Nondairy Milk Alternatives

There is an increasing variety of nondairy milk alternatives available at health-food stores. These include soy milk, soy yogurt, soy cheese, rice milk, soy-rice milk, and nut milks. The broad selection of brands may be overwhelming. Our preferred choice of soy product for taste and versatility in recipes is *Better Than Milk Tofu Soy Beverage*, available in powdered (less expensive) and liquid form. As for soy yogurt and cheese, we aren't too excited about the taste, but both are available. *Rice Dream* is a liquid rice milk made from brown rice, safflower oil, and salt. It does not contain the calcium or protein that complements grain protein as does soy milk. Nut milks are more expensive and too high in fat for some people, but can be a nutritious milk alternative. Of the nut milks, almond milk will provide the

best source of calcium. Recipes for soy yogurt and nut milk
are available in **Eating Better Breakfasts** (see p. 384).

Cheeses

Cheese is an excellent food, but hard cheeses are very
high in fat except for a few. Mozzarella cheese is the best
known and most widely available. It contains half the fat
content of cheddar cheeses. We prefer cheeses that do not
have food coloring added. If the cheese is yellow, coloring
has been added. Use natural cheddar cheeses in preference
to processed American cheeses. Small amounts of Parmesan and Romano cheeses are good choices, especially
freshly grated. Both ricotta and low-fat cottage cheese are
lower in fat than hard cheeses. Nonfat cottage cheese is
readily available, as well, and pleasing to most tastes. All
cheeses have quite a bit of sodium in them unless otherwise
labeled "low" or "no" sodium.

What About Calcium?

If you do not use dairy products, sufficient calcium may
be obtained in other ways. Check *Best Food Sources for Vitamins and Minerals* (p. 142) for other good calcium food
sources, or tack the handy calcium chart at the end of this
chapter on your refrigerator. For women past menopause,
calcium may be of particular concern to reduce loss of bone
mass (osteoporosis), although many studies have not been
conclusive that higher amounts of calcium will accomplish
this purpose. Low estrogen may be more involved with this
loss. However, 1000 mg. of calcium daily is recommended
for post-menopausal women who take estrogen hormone
and 1500 mg. for those who do not. In this case, a good
calcium supplement may be desired. It is wise to do a little
research before choosing a calcium supplement. We recommend *Bone Builder* as a first choice. *Bone Builder* is demarrowed
whole bone concentrate taken from young New Zealand cattle.
It is designated by the scientific term MCHC (Microcrystalline

Hydroxyapatite Concentrate). Scientific studies show that MCHC is a highly absorbable calcium with other important supporting minerals that can increase bone density, and even help to restore lost bone. In contrast, other forms of calcium supplements have been shown in most cases to slow bone loss, but not stop it. Better choices of other calcium supplement sources include calcium citrate or calcium in combination with magnesium (these minerals should be in balance with twice as much calcium as magnesium). *Bone Builder* and other calcium supplements are available at health-food stores. Calcium supplements are best taken with food and not more than 600 mg. at a time.

The amount of calcium available to the body is also influenced by other food habits. Excessive protein (particularly meat protein), refined sugars, and caffeine, for example, draw calcium out of the body, while foods rich in vitamins A, C, D, and zinc (such as dairy, eggs, legumes, and fish), will assist in calcium assimilation. The mineral boron, available in apples, also assists calcium absorption. Again, many things work together for or against health.

Conclusion

Weston A. Price, D.D.S., reports in his book *Nutrition and Physical Degeneration*: "The most physically perfect people in northern India are probably the Pathans who live on dairy products largely in the form of soured curd, together with wheat and vegetables."[8] Perhaps many of the problems of eating dairy products have more to do with what modern food technology has done to them. According to the *Eating Better Lifestyle* chart (p. 39) you can see that the emphasis of our diet is not placed on dairy products in the forms available to us in the United States.

Summary of Dairy Product Choices
Milk
goat's milk
raw certified milk—whole, nonfat, or a combination

raw certified kefir
plain yogurt, whole pasteurized (not homogenized) with
  active cultures
plain yogurt, nonfat or low-fat with active cultures
buttermilk (available at ½%, 1%, 1½%, 2% fat)
nonfat (skim milk)

With caution: low-fat milk yogurt prepared with homogenized whole milk

Avoid: homogenized whole milk

Nondairy Alternatives
soy milk (especially *Better Than Milk Tofu Soy Beverage*)
soy yogurt
soy-rice milk
rice milk (e.g. *Rice Dream*)
nut milks (especially almond)

Cheeses

natural cheeses with no food coloring (raw certified,
  if available)
mozzarella cheese
Parmesan and Romano cheese (especially fresh)
nonfat or low-fat cottage cheese (raw certified, if available)
skim milk ricotta cheese
low sodium and reduced fat types without food coloring

Avoid: processed cheese and cheese foods

Cooking Recommendation: Heat milk as little as possible.
Bring just to a boil when necessary. Use cultured milks
(buttermilk, yogurt) in preference to sweet milk in baking.
Powdered buttermilk is available at health-food stores.
Darigold is a commonly available brand.

Emilie's Cheese Storage Hints:

Soft, ripened cheeses such as brie and camembert freeze
well; wrap tightly. It is best to freeze whole wheels or large

pieces. Semi-hard and hard cheeses such as cheddar will slice poorly and will crumble once frozen.

Two cubes of sugar stored with any cheese in an airtight container will help to retard the growth of mold.

All cheeses are more flavorful at room temperature than when cold. However, hard cheeses are easier to slice while still cold.

Sue's Cheese Hints for Cooking

When cheese is to be melted, pre-grated cheese from the freezer can be a welcome last-minute time-saver. Grate several cups at a time, divide in desired portions, and freeze in Ziploc freezer bags.

Add cheese to dishes just before serving, when possible, and heat just until melted. The more protein is "cooked," the harder it is to digest.

Good Calcium Food Sources

Dairy
1 c. nonfat milk—316 mg.
1 c. low-fat milk—352 mg.
1 c. whole milk—290 mg.
1/4 c. nonfat milk powder—377 mg.
1 c. nonfat yogurt—350 mg.
1 c. low-fat yogurt—415 mg.
1 c. buttermilk—300 mg.
1 c. nonfat cottage cheese—350 mg.
1 c. low-fat cottage cheese—415 mg.
1/4 c. cheddar cheese—205 mg.

Green Vegetables
1 c. cooked broccoli—178 mg.
1 c. cooked beet greens—164 mg.
1/2 c. cooked spinach—122 mg.
2 cups raw spinach—112 mg.
1/2 c. bok choy—79 mg.
   (Chinese cabbage)
1/2 c. cooked collard greens—74 mg.
1/2 c. cooked dandelion greens—73 mg.
1/2 c. raw dandelion greens—52 mg.
1/2 c. cooked okra—50 mg.

Soy/Legumes
1 c. Tofu Soy Beverage—400 mg.
   (Better Than Milk brand)
1 c. cooked soybeans—131 mg.
1/2 c. cooked legumes—25–60 mg.

Fish
1/2 c. salmon—239 mg.
4 oz. red snapper—45 mg.

Nuts/Seeds
1 c. almond milk—83 mg.
1/4 c. sesame seeds—351 mg.
1/4 c. sunflower seeds—42 mg.

Misc.
1 tbsp. blackstrap molasses—140 mg.
1 tbsp. carob powder—31 mg.

Recommended Daily Dietary
Allowances—Calcium

 800 mg.—children, 1–10; males, over 18; females, 24 to menopause
1200 mg.—males, 11–18; females, 11–18; pregnant/lactating women
1000 mg.—post-menopausal women on estrogen hormone
1500 mg.—post-menopausal women not on estrogen hormone

25

Those Magnificent Micronutrients

———— ♥ ————

I will give you the treasures of darkness, riches stored in secret places, so that you may know that I am the LORD.

Isaiah 45:3

———— ♥ ————

*V*itamins interact in thousands of ways with enzymes to carry on all body processes, while minerals are an integral part of all body tissue and involved in many body processes as well. Each vitamin and mineral performs so many life-giving functions that they are truly a great wonder of our Lord's creative genius and power! We cannot possibly list the many tasks of the micronutrients in such a short space. The *Nutrition Almanac* is an excellent reference on vitamins and minerals.

The fact that the first vitamin was not discovered until as recently as 1886 ought to arouse skepticism about the completeness of synthetic vitamins, either in tablet form or in refined foods fortified with them. Persons who insist that the body does not know the difference between synthetic and natural vitamins overlook the probability of unknown nutrients contained in the natural forms. Whole foods will best supply what is yet undiscovered.

Prevention of deficiency diseases such as beriberi, pellagra, anemia, or scurvy is not a good measure of adequate vitamin and mineral intake. It is this view that fostered the enrichment of white flour with vitamins B_1, B_2, B_3, and iron. We now know that the complete range of micronutrients is vital in our resistance to illnesses, degenerative diseases, and premature aging. Americans by the millions are suffering marginal vitamin and mineral deficiencies fostered by the refined food diet. For example, the loss of vitamin E in white flour is 86%, yet vitamin E plays a key role in the prevention of heart disease. The implication is that millions suffer from heart disease not only because of high fat intake but also from vitamin E deficiency. This means that our supply of vitamins and minerals in whole foods is just as vital to health and disease prevention as are low fat and high fiber.

The only way to guarantee the complete micronutrient package is to eat a varied diet of whole foods. It is not necessary or practical to count micrograms or milligrams of vitamins and minerals to make sure you are getting enough. A varied diet of whole foods that provides enough calories, protein, carbohydrates, and fat will usually provide all the vitamins and minerals you can get from food. While many persons in America may also need to support the diet with additional vitamin and mineral supplements, all need the foundation of the *Eating Better Lifestyle*.

The *Best Food Sources of Vitamins and Minerals* list begins on page 138. This will guide you in choosing the variety of foods that supply them. Keep in mind that vitamins and minerals are widely distributed throughout all foods. You will receive small amounts from many varied food sources.

Water-soluble vitamins, the B-vitamins, and vitamin C are washed out of the body daily and, therefore, must be replenished daily. Fat-soluble vitamins and minerals can be stored in the body. It is almost impossible to get an overdose of any vitamin or mineral from eating a variety of whole foods.

Vitamin A in animal foods and plant foods is not the same. True "preformed" vitamin A (called retinol) is found only in animal foods, and is considered completely absorbable by the human body. All vitamin A from plant sources is "provitamin A" (called carotene) and is only partially absorbed by the body. The body must convert carotene into vitamin A before it can be utilized as vitamin A. To date, the adult RDA of vitamin A is set at 5000 I.U. (International Units). This level is based on an expected intake of half retinol vitamin A from animal foods, and half carotene, provitamin A, from plant foods. If no animal foods are eaten, more than the equivalent of 5000 I.U. of vitamin A must be consumed in plant foods to obtain the RDA allowance. The Recommended Daily Allowances set by the USDA, by the way, are based on minimal health requirements, not necessarily what is needed for optimum health. There is, thankfully, an abundance of plant foods high in provitamin A (see p. 139).

Proper food storage and preparation will affect the availability of vitamins and minerals. In general, vitamin C and the B-vitamins are the most perishable, easily destroyed by air, heat, moisture, and light. To preserve vitamin C and other nutrients, store foods (except those with protective skins) in closed containers. Store most fresh foods—except those with protective skins that need to ripen at room temperature (e.g. bananas, cantaloupe, tomatoes)—in well-covered containers and away from light in the refrigerator.

The best storage containers for fresh produce are those that let out moisture and the gases that speed up ripening, while preserving the nutrients. We recommend *Evert-Fresh Bags*, available nationwide in some drug stores, kitchen specialty shops, and supermarkets. Evert-Fresh Bags are impregnated with processed Oya stone from caves in Japan where produce has been successfully stored for three centuries. Oya stone has the ability to absorb the ethylene gas given off by produce that accelerates aging and deterioration. In addition, the permeability of Evert-Fresh Bags allows the discharge of other gases such as ammonia and carbon dioxide. These bags are also treated to minimize moisture formation, inhibiting mold and bacteria growth. Up to 50% of the vitamin C may be preserved by using Evert-Fresh Bags. If you cannot locate these, see p. 305. These reusable green bags are available in small, medium, and large sizes in packages of 10.

Ziploc Vegetable Bags are now also available in gallon and pint size in supermarkets for fresh produce storage. These have freshness vents that release the right amount of moisture to protect freshness. Store fresh foods away from light in the refrigerator or in cold storage.

Eat many fruits and vegetables raw and do not wash or cut them until ready to eat, except leafy greens (see chapter 27). Cook vegetables lightly, just until crisp-tender. Quick stir-fry or steaming will preserve nutrients the best. If you boil vegetables, use only a very small amount of water. The exception is broccoli (p. 362). Save the cooking water to use in soups, breads, and bean or grain dishes. Keep a covered jar handy to store leftover vegetable water in the refrigerator.

An excellent reference to whole-food storage is *Keeping Food Fresh* by Janet Bailey.

Best Food Sources of Vitamins and Minerals

Vitamin A (fat soluble)
  o.g.* liver of beef, lamb, poultry, cheeses, eggs, whole milk, halibut, mackerel, fish liver oil

---

* Organically grown. Liver can be very toxic if not organically grown. For a definition of organically grown, see p. 187.

Provitamin A (carotene) (fat soluble)

vegetables: all dark leafy greens (spinach, kale, beet greens, collards, chard, mustard greens, sorrel, turnip greens, dandelion greens, lamb's-quarters), dark yellow vegetables (carrots, sweet potatoes, yams [U.S. variety], yellow squash, pumpkin), broccoli, endive, arugula, loose-leaf lettuce, romaine lettuce, red peppers, tomatoes, parsley, rutabagas, brussels sprouts, green beans, asparagus, lima beans, green peas, sweet corn

fruits: apricots, cantaloupe, sour cherries, mangoes, nectarines, papaya, peaches, persimmons, watermelon

Vitamin C (water soluble)

vegetables: dark leafy greens (collards, kale, spinach, mustard greens, turnip greens, sorrel, lamb's-quarters), broccoli, cabbage, green and red peppers, okra, green peas, brussels sprouts, parsley, Irish potatoes, sweet potatoes, yams (U.S. variety), cauliflower, tomatoes

fruits: citrus (oranges, grapefruit, tangerines, lemons, limes), kiwi fruit, pineapple, papaya, mangoes, berries (strawberries, loganberries, blackberries, raspberries), guava, honeydew melon, cantaloupe

Vitamin D (fat soluble)
fish liver oil (cod, halibut), sardines, herring, salmon, tuna, egg yolks, fortified milk

Vitamin E (fat soluble)
whole grains, vegetable oils (unrefined or cold-pressed safflower, soybean, corn), soybeans, eggs, dark leafy greens, broccoli, brussels sprouts, cabbage, asparagus, raw nuts and seeds, peanuts

Vitamin K (fat soluble)
yogurt, egg yolks, beef, blackstrap molasses, vegetable oils (sunflower, safflower, soybean), fish liver oils, kelp,

leafy green vegetables (cabbage, kale, spinach), green peas, carrots, cauliflower, tomatoes—and the human body can make vitamin K

Vitamin P (biflavonoids or C complex) (water soluble)
white skins of citrus fruits, apricots, buckwheat, green peppers, tomatoes, apricots, rhubarb, blackberries, cherries, rose hips

Essential Fatty Acids (linoleic, linolenic, arachidonic)
vegetable oils (sunflower, safflower, soybean, peanut), wheat germ in whole wheat, sunflower seeds, walnuts, pecans, almonds, avocados—and the human body can make linolenic and arachidonic (if enough linoleic is present), flaxseed oil, canola oil

B-Vitamins (water soluble)
B-vitamins generally are present together in the same foods; whole grains, eggs, leafy greens

B_1 *(thiamine)*
whole grains, peanuts, beef kidney, milk, eggs, plums, prunes, raisins, blackstrap molasses

B_2 *(riboflavin)*
milk; o.g. liver, kidney, and heart of lamb, beef, veal; cheese, green vegetables, broccoli, eggs

B_3 *(niacin)*
whole grains; o.g. liver of beef, chicken, veal, and lamb; eggs, lean meat, poultry, fish (swordfish, tuna, halibut), roasted peanuts, dates, figs, avocados, prunes—and the human body can make niacin

B_6 *(pyridoxine)*
whole rye flour, brown rice, buckwheat (kasha), whole wheat; o.g. liver and heart; chicken, beef, eggs, cantaloupe, cabbage, blackstrap molasses, fish (herring, mackerel, salmon), peanuts, soybeans, walnuts

B_{12} *(cobalamin)*
milk; o.g. liver of lamb, beef; veal, egg yolks, fish (herring, salmon, sardines)

B_{13} *(orotic acid)*
whey (cultured dairy), root vegetables

B_{15} *(pangamic acid)*
whole grains, brown rice, pumpkin seeds, sesame seeds, o.g. liver

B_{17} *(laetrile) (amygdalin)*
whole grains, legumes (dry beans), wild berries, kernels of apricots, apples, cherries, peaches, plums, nectarines, cashews, macadamia nuts, sprouts (alfalfa, mung, garbanzo, wheat), unhulled sesame seeds, flax seeds, chia seeds

Biotin
wheat, milk, o.g. beef liver, egg yolks, chicken, salmon, brown rice, nuts, fruits, corn, mushrooms—and the human body can make biotin

Pantothenic Acid
wheat, eggs; o.g. liver, kidney and heart of beef, chicken, and lamb; green vegetables, herring, whole grains, nuts, raw peanuts

Choline
wheat; o.g. beef liver, heart, and brain; leafy green vegetables, peanuts

Folic Acid
whole wheat, dark leafy greens, egg yolks; o.g. liver of beef, lamb, and chicken; tuna, cantaloupe, asparagus, carrots, apricots, pumpkins, avocados, beans, dark rye flour

Inositol
whole wheat; o.g. beef heart, liver, and brain; cantaloupe, cabbage, raisins, dried limas, grapefruit—and the human body can make inositol

PABA *(para-aminobenzoic acid)*
   whole grains, brown rice, liver, kidney, molasses, yogurt—and the human body can make PABA

Calcium
   milk, cheeses, cottage cheese, yogurt, sardines, salmon,
   cooked leafy green vegetables (beet greens, spoon cabbage, chard, kale, collards, mustard greens, turnip
   greens, dandelion greens, lamb's-quarters), broccoli,
   okra, dried beans, unhulled sesame seeds, blackstrap
   molasses, carob, rhubarb

Chlorine
   salt, kelp, dulse, plant seafood, rye flour, ripe olives

Chromium
   meat, chicken, corn oil, brewer's yeast (supplement)

Cobalt
   meat, kidney, liver, milk, plant seafood

Copper
   leafy green vegetables, dried beans, peas, whole grains,
   prunes, almonds, most seafood, calf and beef liver

Fluorine
   seafoods, gelatin

Iodine
   kelp, onions, plant seafood, fish, vegetables grown in
   iodine-rich soil (especially mushrooms); table salt is not
   a good source (see pp. 190-91)

Iron
   beef liver, heart, kidney; lean red meat, dried peaches,
   egg yolks, nuts, beans, asparagus, blackstrap molasses,
   oatmeal, leafy green vegetables

Magnesium
   figs, lemons, grapefruit, apples, green vegetables, yellow corn, soybeans, wheat, almonds, nuts, seeds

Manganese
  leafy green vegetables, peas, beets, nuts, whole grains, egg yolks

Molybdenum
  dark leafy green vegetables, whole grains, legumes

Phosphorus
  fish, poultry, meat, whole grains, eggs, nuts, seeds

Potassium
  citrus fruits, watercress, all green leafy vegetables, mint leaves, sunflower seeds, bananas, potatoes (especially peelings), oranges, whole grains

Selenium
  whole wheat, tuna fish, onions, broccoli, tomatoes

Sodium
  salt, carrots, beets, artichokes, kelp, seafoods, poultry, meat

Sulfur
  brussels sprouts, cabbage, dried beans, nuts, eggs, fish, lean beef

Vanadium
  fish

Zinc
  whole grains, eggs, ground mustard, round steak, lamb chops, pumpkin seeds, brewer's yeast (supplement)

26

The Sensation of Sugar

———— ♥ ————

*Eat honey, my son, for it is good. . . . If you find honey,
eat just enough. . . . It is not good to eat too much
honey.*

Proverbs 24:13; 25:16,27

———— ♥ ————

*W*hy do we seek out sweet foods? When man gathered foods from the wild, sweet plants were usually safe in contrast to the bitter which were often poisonous. It was probably man's instinct for the sweet taste that led him to seek out sweet fruits containing choice nutrients such as vitamin C and natural quick-energy-producing sugars. It is not our inherited drive for sweet things that is at fault. It is the many refined food products that retain the sweetness but not the nutrients. Food companies know that we love them and, therefore, spend $400 million yearly to advertise foods on television. Half of them are sweet foods.

Sugar was first cultivated in India in 325 B.C., but remained a scarce luxury for many centuries. It became a common food only in the last 100 years. By the 1980s the average yearly sugar consumption in America had reached about 120 lbs. per person—over 500 calories per day. In the 1990s sugar consumption has come down somewhat, much of it due no doubt to the availability of food products sweetened with *NutraSweet*. Food manufacturers continue to produce a wide variety of new sweets to feed our inherent desire for them!

Not all will agree that refined sugar is death in the pot, yet its effects on health have been extensively researched. Sugar has been implicated in the following effects on bodily health:

- Increased blood cholesterol and triglyceride levels that contribute to heart disease

- Unstable blood sugar levels that contribute to hypoglycemia, diabetes, and aggravate criminal behavior

- Depletion of B-vitamins stored in the body which contributes to depression, an intensified craving for alcohol in alcoholics, and excessive estrogen in women that contributes to breast cancer.[1]

- Displacement of more nutritious foods with empty calories contributing to obesity, and lowered resistance to most health problems and degenerative diseases

- Upset of the homeostasis (balance) mechanism which causes a perpetual craving for sugar—sugar addiction

- Increased uric acid in the blood leading to gout

- Reduction of phosphorus in the blood that prevents bone calcification, and leaching of calcium from the bones that contributes to osteoporosis

♥ Altered pH (acid/base) balance in the mouth which causes tooth decay

♥ Reduced effectiveness of white blood cells to kill bacteria, thus encouraging infections

What are some ways to reduce refined sugar consumption? What are the alternatives? If we lived on a sugar plantation, we could chew on sugarcane, a whole-food nutrient package. Chewing on sugarcane is not the same as consuming white sugar from which all the original fiber and nutrients are extracted. Fresh fruits, our best sources of natural sweets, are widely available. They are truly God's desserts requiring little or no preparation. Nevertheless, most of us want some sweetening to cook with, too. What is the best?

Our first choice is honey. The biblical record for honey sets aside the argument that honey is no better than refined sugar. God's Word is especially clear about this particular food: "Eat honey, my son, for it is good . . . but not too much." We wonder if God had the twentieth century in mind! He created honey as a whole, natural food with a wealth of nutritional value, minute as the amounts may be. Arguments that these amounts are too small to count are presumptuous. Besides, God gave the Israelites "a land flowing with milk and honey." Would He expect them not to eat the honey? Its goodness is extolled by those who have learned to appreciate it:

> Containing 39 percent fructose, honey is an important antifatigue food. Since it is predigested, it builds up alkaline reserves in the blood and tissues, and provides a maximum of energy with a minimum of shock to the digestive system. Sugar-laden foods overload the bloodstream in 15 minutes; honey is absorbed over a period of four hours.

> There is no energy-producing food on the market to touch honey. Nor will there ever be. All

synthetic glucose products are inferior to honey, not only for the speed with which they bring about a sense of well-being, but also for the production of real lasting energy and the alkalinizing of the body.[2]

Honey contains minute amounts of a wealth of nutrients including B-vitamins, vitamin C, and at least 12 minerals. It has many other nutrient properties not fully understood, including bee pollen protein of high value. Honey is easily and rapidly assimilated, provides a natural, gentle laxative effect, and is easier on the kidneys to process than all other sugars. The nutrients in honey assist in its partial digestion. When combined with whole-grain flour or cereal high in dietary fiber and B-vitamins, the body can digest honey very well without depleting stored nutrients.

We must also heed the biblical warning not to eat too much honey. Start by reducing the number of desserts and sweets. Sugar intake can be reduced further by using half as much honey as white sugar in recipes, since it is twice as sweet. The strong flavor curbs appetite, too. The flavor depends on what flowers the bees visited to collect nectar. Lighter honey is usually a milder flavor. You may prefer a milder honey for puddings and toppings, but a darker honey works well in baking. Like olive oil, honey is an expensive ingredient. This hidden blessing will also limit our use of it!

As with other good foods, honey can be refined. Heating over 160° and straining removes valuable bee pollen and some of the nutrients. Supermarket honey and much of it in health-food stores is refined. The best quality honey is unheated, unfiltered honey. Honey labeled "uncooked" does not classify as "unheated" because it can be heated to 160° and still be labeled "uncooked." Top-quality honey is a very expensive health-food-store item. Purchasing honey in five-gallon cans from a local beekeeper will be the least expensive. Honey can be stored indefinitely. If supermarket honey is the only honey available to you, use it as a first step to breaking the refined sugar habit.

Since heating honey destroys some of its nutritional value, heat it as little as possible when cooking over direct heat, adding it toward the last of the cooking process. When honey is used in baking, it is protected somewhat by being combined with other ingredients.

Although honey is our first choice, there are other alternatives to white sugar. Among others, these include pure maple syrup, blackstrap molasses, sorghum, date sugar, and crystalline or liquid fructose. All of these are expensive and not as widely available as honey. The health-food store is the best place to find them. Pure maple syrup has a good amount of potassium and calcium. Don't confuse it with supermarket pancake syrup that is made with white sugar or corn syrup and imitation maple flavoring. Pure maple syrup comes from maple trees. Use it occasionally for pancakes and waffles. Sorghum is high in calcium, phosphorus, riboflavin, niacin, and iron. Blackstrap molasses contains most of the nutrients refined out of white sugar. It is high in calcium, potassium, and iron. It has a stronger flavor and more nutrient value than the light and dark molasses sold in supermarkets. Date sugar, actually ground dates, is high in potassium, B-vitamins, and vitamin A. Fructose, derived primarily from corn, contains little nutrient value. Its two advantages over white sugar are that it requires less release of insulin in the body and, like honey, requires about half the amount in most recipes, even though it is not quite twice as sweet as sugar. We use it only in an occasional recipe, such as angel food cake, where honey really does not work very well, or when a very small amount of sugar is needed—in a salad dressing, for example. Crystalline fructose is interchangeable with honey in most recipes.

Until recently whole sugarcane was not available in the United States. Now, however, an excellent whole cane sugar is being marketed in health food stores called Sucanat (an abbreviation of SUgarCAne NATural). Sucanat is evaporated whole sugarcane juice, continuing its full range of nutrients. The rich nutrient value of molasses is included in Sucanat. We have been pleased with the results of Sucanat in baking. It is a good alternative for honey, giving variation in flavor and texture. It has restored some of the desired crispness in cookies while honey and fructose produce cookies that are cake-like in texture. We have introduced the use of Sucanat in *Eating Better Desserts* (see p. 384). Try the *Orange or Lemon Spice Cookies* (see p. 369) with Sucanat. We use the same amount of Sucanat to replace white sugar and twice as much to replace honey. Sucanat, cup for cup, costs about the same as honey. Unfortunately it costs twice as much to use (1 cup Sucanat to ½ cup honey). Nevertheless, it is less expensive than several other natural sweeteners, including date sugar, maple syrup, and fruit concentrates.

Fruit concentrates have come into use in the 1990s in many commercial products. Growing awareness of these has aroused an interest in using them in home baking. We have introduced, for example, the use of Mystic Lake Dairy Sweetener in *Desserts*. This sweetener consists of 100% pineapple syrup, pear and peach juice concentrates. Many health-food stores carry it. It replaces 1 cup sugar or ½ cup honey or fructose and often eliminates the need for added fat.

All of these sugars are combinations of the simple sugars— fructose, glucose, maltose, and sucrose. Fresh fruits, fruit juices, high fructose corn syrup, and honey are highest in fructose. Maltose is the form of sugar primarily in milk and beer. Molasses, Sucanat, white and brown sugar, maple syrup, raw and turbinado sugar, and sorghum are all primarily sucrose. Refined sugars used in prepackaged foods include high fructose corn syrup, corn syrup solids, dextrose, dextrins, invert sugar, sucrose, and glucose. A most effective way to remove refined sugars from the diet is to replace prepackaged foods with basic whole foods. In addition there are many prepackaged foods in health-food stores that do not contain refined sugars—such as those sweetened with a fruit concentrate.

What about artificial sweeteners such as saccharin, cyclamates, Equal, NutraSweet, and aspartame? The history of saccharin and cyclamates should suggest to us that the current unchecked use of aspartame in hundreds of food products is not a guaranteed measure of its boon to health. Aspartame, also known as Equal and NutraSweet, has been pronounced safe by the Federal Food and Drug Administration. The FDA has undoubtedly been pressured by large food businesses that wish to use aspartame in many products. In the meantime, many news articles have appeared that report concern about the effects of aspartame, especially in regard to brain chemistry. Problematic effects from aspartame seem most likely to occur when several cans of soda pop with aspartame are consumed with carbohydrates such as a sandwich or a candy bar. There is also some concern that aspartame may adversely affect the unborn baby. We do not have sufficient information about aspartame to make a wise judgment. We suggest caution in using Equal, or food products containing aspartame and NutraSweet, and that pregnant women avoid them altogether. A short review of aspartame's history is presented in *A Consumer Dictionary of Food Additives* by Ruth Winter (see Recommended Reading, p. 379). Finally, we may ask the question, "Can man develop any imitation food that equals the nutritional lifegiving value of God's original whole foods?"

What is the sugarholic to do? There is hope! If you are addicted to sugar, there are several things you can do to break the habit. A frequent protein snack such as an egg, piece of cheese, or plain yogurt may help. Protein can curb a sugar craving by stabilizing the blood sugar level. Eating several small snacks throughout the day of fresh fruit, nuts, seeds, or raw vegetables can help. All of these contain natural sugars that will produce a slow rise in blood sugar level. Many people are especially helped by eating nuts and seeds. Try unsalted and unroasted sunflower seeds. They are the least expensive. Soaking sunflower seeds or almonds in water for two to eight hours before eating them will improve digestibility. Soaked sunflower seeds have a very pleasing crunch. Nuts and seeds must be chewed very well to digest properly. Blending a few of them in protein shakes will help, too. An increase in unrefined complex carbohydrate foods that are high in B-vitamins (such as breads and cereals) also will decrease the sugar craving. You may enjoy eating whole-grain muffins in place of sugary foods. The honey content is much lower than in cakes, cookies, and desserts. Try *Minute Blender Bran Muffins* (p. 356), and especially *Emilie's Deluxe Bran Muffins* (p. 357). Try fruit shakes with no additional sugar such as *Sunshine Shake* (p. 364), *Orange Frosty* (p. 365), and *Fruit Smoothie* (p. 366). You can blend shakes up in a matter of minutes, not only for a satisfying "sweet treat," but also for a nutrient-rich "complete meal in a glass."*

Honey Tips

Cooking with Honey: Reduce oven temperature by 25° when substituting honey for white or brown sugar in any favorite recipe.

Honey for Babies? Wait until baby has passed the first birthday before feeding honey. Botulism spores may be in honey and are potentially dangerous for infants under one year. There is no known danger to anyone older. Furthermore, there is no point in introducing any kind of concentrated sugar to a baby.

Emilie's Beauty Aid: I clean my face, then put honey all over it and relax 10–15 minutes—rinse well. Smooth, soft skin appears.

More muffin and shake recipes are available in the *Eating Better Cookbooks*. See pp. 383-84 for information.

27

Raw Foods in Review

———— ♥ ————

On each side of the river stood the tree of life, bearing twelve crops of fruit, yielding its fruit every month. And the leaves of the tree are for the healing of the nations.

Revelation 22:2

———— ♥ ————

The *Eating Better Lifestyle* includes lots of raw fruits and vegetables. No vitamins and minerals are lost in cooking. Their high content of pure water assists in cleansing waste products from the body. Chlorophyll in green plants is also very cleansing for the bloodstream.

Nutritionists do not agree on the benefit of plant enzymes to the human body, but many believe that they are vital to human health. Some even claim that raw foods are the only kind that mankind should eat because all enzymes are destroyed by cooking. Whether or not our bodies need the enzymes, raw foods have enough advantages to warrant a favored place in our diet.

It is unlikely that many Americans would adopt an all-raw-foods diet on a long-term basis, but a short-term diet of all raw food for a week or two can help to rejuvenate the body. It might be good to know that if you lose your cooking facilities or fuel, you can thrive on raw foods. You can also sprout seeds, grains, and beans. Vitamins and minerals are multiplied many times from the original seed, bean, or grain when grown into sprouts. The protein value of sprouts is also excellent.

It is easy to grow alfalfa sprouts. Soak two tablespoons of alfalfa seeds from a health-food store in a quart jar covered with a piece of screen held in place with a rubber band. Soak overnight, drain, and tip the jar downward in a bowl on your kitchen counter. Water the sprouts once every morning and evening, keeping them well drained. In five to seven days your jar will be full of fresh sprouts to use in sandwiches and salads or to snack on. Cover them tightly and refrigerate. They will keep up to two weeks. For the value of their nutrition, sprouts are the most inexpensive food. They are also free of pesticides.

There is nothing like vine-ripened fresh produce for nutrition and flavor. Garden growing provides a wonderful opportunity and is often our only chance to get fresh food grown without pesticides. Eat the edible peelings on fruits and vegetables as much as possible because much of the nutrient content is near the surface. Recycle your produce scraps in the compost pile. Your garbage disposal doesn't need them! For information on storing fresh produce, see pp. 137-38.

Several products are available to clean fruits and vegetables: Amway L.O.C., Shaklee Basic-H, Dr. Donsbach's Superoxy Food Wash (advertised to reduce pesticide residues, food waxes, and many harmful chemicals), and Nature Clean All Purpose Cleaning Lotion (a Canadian product new to the United States). Look in health-food stores for the two latter products. If you cannot find them, see p. 306.

To wash greens and leafy greens such as lettuce, broccoli, brussels sprouts, and parsley, fill the sink with water. Immerse the vegetables two or more times as needed to thoroughly rinse, changing the water after each rinse. An additional rinse under running water, leaf by leaf, is often needed for lettuce. Spin the water out of leafy greens. We do not wash or cut fresh produce until just before preparing them to eat (to retain nutrients and minimize moisture in storage) except for leafy greens that will be eaten fresh. The reason for this is that washing and drying lettuce for salad at the last minute is a tedious job and is therefore not likely to be done well.

Avoid buying potatoes that have a greenish tinge. The discoloration is caused by prolonged exposure to light, developing a toxic poison called solanine and giving the potatoes a slightly bitter taste. If you must use such potatoes, peel them and trim away all the green part. Store potatoes properly in a dark, humid, well-ventilated place at a cool 45-50°. You can store them in the refrigerator if needed.

28

A Salty Sermon

♥

Salt is good.   Luke 14:34

Is tasteless food eaten without salt . . . ? I refuse to touch it; such food makes me ill.

                                                                Job 6:6,7

♥

The American Diet averages 4000 to 6000 milligrams of sodium per day. The Recommended Dietary Allowance is 2400 milligrams per day. The *Eating Better Lifestyle* menus and recipes allow you to use salt in cooking and baking, yet within the 2400 milligram range.* Below this range, taste becomes an obstacle to many people. Actually, the human body requires less than 500 milligrams of sodium per day which can be obtained from our food without the addition of salt. Learning to season food well without salt

---

* The "no salt" diet is a therapeutic diet (see p. 53). The *Eating Better Lifestyle* is not a therapeutic diet, although recipes and menus are adaptable with specific modifications.

requires skill and practice. The following guidelines will help to curb the sodium level without eliminating salt altogether:

- ♥ Leave salt off the table.

- ♥ Do not salt vegetables while cooking.

- ♥ Save the salt for baking and main dishes or other flavorful recipes such as soups. Season to taste to reduce original amount called for.

- ♥ Use low-sodium baking powder in baking (available at health-food stores).

- ♥ Use soy sauce reduced in sodium. Kikkoman Lite or Milder (Lite is considerably less expensive; persons allergic to wheat should not use Kikkoman).

- ♥ Use *Sue's "Kitchen Magic"* seasoning in place of chicken bouillon (see p. 383).

With the freedom to use a little salt, the taste of whole foods—especially grains and beans—will go from bland to delightful.

Purchase a higher-quality salt with trace minerals and containing neither aluminum nor dextrose and which has not been kiln dried. Most of these salts are labeled as sea salt, but not all sea salts are of the same quality. Look for the label "sun evaporated only" or for "unheated" salt. We recommend RealSalt. (See p. 304 for mail-order information.)

A reduction from 6000 mg. or more of sodium in the diet to 2400 mg. or less is a great improvement and quite adequate for most people. In order to do this, of course, you will need to omit most packaged foods with salt added. But do not be overly concerned about using canned tomato products or tuna fish unless you make dishes with them every day. They are both very high in sodium, but you can still use some in cooking. Tomato paste is much lower than tomato sauce in sodium. We are also finding canned tomatoes on the supermarket shelves with no salt, so check the labels carefully. Lemon juice added to unsalted tuna compensates for the lack of salt. Start with 50%-salt-reduced tuna.

Canned beans (legumes) are also very high in sodium, whereas dry beans contain little. "No salt added" or "50% reduced salt" canned beans are available. The sodium content of canned beans can be reduced up to 40% by draining off all the juice and rinsing them thoroughly under running water for one minute. Canned beans without salt or dry beans can be used in recipes without increasing the salt added. For cooked beans in salads, canned beans with some salt provide a more pleasing flavor.

High blood pressure is a serious problem. Sixty million persons have it, and many do not even know it. It is the leading cause of strokes and the cause of about 30% of all heart disease. In addition, many overweight persons have a water retention problem. Salt consumption, however, is not the sole cause of high blood pressure and water retention. The lack of calcium in the diet along with accompanying low levels of potassium, vitamin A, and vitamin C may have just as much or more to do with these problems. David A. McCarron, M.D., in *Science* (June 29, 1984) reported the findings of a study involving calcium and high blood pressure. "We've always thought of heart disease in terms of excesses, especially excesses of sodium and cholesterol. . . . But these patterns are patterns of deficiency . . . so let's deal with these deficiencies and step back from hammering on dietary restrictions."[1] This study also demonstrated a correlation between higher consumption of dairy products and lower blood pressure levels. "Increased consumption of dairy products would be associated with a correction in potassium and calcium deficits."[2] Dr. McCarron states that if we consumed at least 800 milligrams of calcium daily (the RDA for the average adult) and 3000 to 3500 milligrams of potassium, "It's likely that sodium will take care of itself."[3]

There is evidence that magnesium levels are also involved. Denise Foley reports in "Foods to Lower Your Blood Pressure," *Prevention* (July 1984, p. 30), "One of the most interesting things to come out of Dr. McCarron's research is not how calcium works alone to lower blood pressure but how it works with potassium, sodium and magnesium to regulate pressure. 'It's the proportions of these minerals in the body that seem to be the most important thing,' says Dr. McCarron." Again we are talking about synergism (things working best in combination) and that is just what a diet of whole food variety provides! We believe this is more important than omitting all salt from cooking. An excellent calcium supplement is *Bone Builder* (see pp. 130-31).

Small amounts of potassium, calcium, and magnesium are widely distributed in whole foods, but some are especially good sources. The chart on pages 138-43 will guide you in choosing these foods. Other findings point to EPA and DHA (also called omega-3 fatty acids) in fish and linoleic acid in polyunsaturated oils as nutrients that contribute to normal blood pressure. High-fiber foods and exercise are also important for normal blood pressure.

29

I'm Sick and Tired of Being Fat!

————— ♥ —————

In the last ten years I have gained 30 diet books and lost 200 lbs.—the same 10 lbs. over and over and over!

————— ♥ —————

Fat is an American obsession. People even die from the fear of it. We call that anorexia and bulimia. We still believe that "fatty, fatty, two by four, can't get through the kitchen door," is a social disgrace! We believe it at the cost of every new diet rage that hits the newsstands. No matter if "diets don't work," we'll try them anyway, again, again, and again! Each new diet proclaims the same sensational promise: "It works!" Yet 95% of 34 million overweight people (25% of the American population) continue to experience the truth of Proverbs 13:12, step A: "Hope deferred makes the heart sick. . . ." We never achieve the hope of step B: "but a longing fulfilled is a tree of life." Witness the following scenario:

Begin new diet, lose weight rapidly for two-
three-four weeks, hit plateau, get discouraged,
hang in there while losing more pounds—more
slowly, reach "ideal" weight—hurrah!, return
to "normal" diet—hungrier than ever, gain
back more pounds than lost on diet! Guilty!
"Must not have done it right. Must gain more
self-control. It couldn't have been the diet, it
must have been me! Maybe I can do better on
the next diet."

Stop! It's time to get off this hopeless diet merry-go-
round and get on the road of hope and health! How are we
going to do that? First we need to understand why low-
calorie dieting fails.

Why Low-Calorie Diets Don't Work

The historical norm is not perpetual feast, but periodic
food shortage and famine. For example, two-thirds of the
world population is currently hungry. There are many biblical accounts of famine such as Genesis 12:10, "Now there
was a famine in the land, and Abram went down to Egypt to
live there for a while because the famine was severe"; Genesis 41:57, "And all the countries came to Egypt to buy grain
from Joseph, because the famine was severe in all the
world"; Ruth 1:1, "In the days when the judges ruled, there
was a famine in the land"; 2 Samuel 21:1, "During the reign
of David, there was a famine for three successive years";
1 Kings 18:2, "Now the famine was severe in Samaria";
Acts 11:28, "One of them, named Agabus, stood up and
through the Spirit predicted that a severe famine would
spread over the entire Roman world"; Matthew 24:7, "There
will be famines and earthquakes in various places."

God designed our bodies to burn fewer calories in times
of food shortage and famine to prolong life on slim pickin's.
How good of Him! Our hope of winning the war on weight
is partially destroyed by low-calorie diets because they create an artificial famine. Therefore, adopting a low-calorie

diet makes it very difficult to return to a normal-calorie level without gaining even more weight back than was lost.

We see Christians struggling to apply spiritual principles to a discipline of dieting that accomplishes just the opposite of what they work and pray for because they are not aware of the way God designed their bodies. The result adds spiritual, emotional, and mental stress, creating volumes of guilt. Our affluence and abundance, an abnormal situation, requires a different approach to weight control than low-calorie dieting.

Step off the diet merry-go-round and forget about all of those low-calorie diets! What a relief! June Bailey thinks so, too. She has written a book called *Fat Is Where It's At*. Bailey has decided to accept herself as she is. "I've learned to like the fat person who lives in this body."[1] She may be going a bit too far in the other direction but many of us need to hear her message about personal worth.

Personal Worth Not Measured in Inches 'n' Pounds

"Your beauty . . . should be that of your inner self, the unfading beauty of a gentle and quiet spirit, which is of great worth in God's sight. For this is the way the holy women of the past who put their hope in God used to make themselves beautiful" (1 Peter 3:3-5). Our friend Helen, though she struggles with being overweight, is a lovely example. We observed her as she demonstrated her professional expertise in producing and directing our video, *"Eating Better with Sue."* When she is not producing and editing films, she is caring for her lively twin nine-year-old boys, caring for her hardworking husband, leading Inner Development groups, and hostessing a popular radio talk show. She radiates the love of Christ in her relationships. Her inner beauty comes through her eyes, her smile, her conversation, and her touch, and it is this that dominates her outward appearance. This is the kind of beauty that God looks for. It is the unseen that is eternal. It is not that

God is disinterested in someone's struggle with obesity. But He does not measure personal worth by it. If this is not your view of yourself, stop now and pray for God's sense of your worth without reference to your body size. As you gain this frame of mind, you can lose your taste for the next fad diet and pursue the *Eating Better Lifestyle* with a gentle and quiet spirit.

Focus on Total Health

Obesity is seldom, if ever, an isolated health problem. When one focuses on weight loss, calories become more important than the total nutrient value of food. For example, low-calorie diet products and recipes frequently contain ingredients of inferior nutritional quality. In addition, it is not easy to get the full Recommended Dietary Allowances of food nutrients on a 1500-calorie diet. Success depends on a permanent lifestyle change in eating habits rather than temporary change. Instead of thinking "fewer calories to lose weight," think, "total nutritional value for total health." Helen, for example, has decided to approach eating in this way. The result is a new focus—not upon her own individual need, but upon the health needs of her entire family.

Watch for a shift in emphasis in the 1990s from weight control to a "total health" approach by some of the organizations that have for many years focused primarily on weight control. Chris wrote to me, "In my previous letter I wrote about a diet program I had joined that was too expensive for me to continue along with the fact my husband wasn't too pleased with the $45 weekly fee. I enclosed two cookbooks I had used during the short time I was on the program. I have no intention of ever going back to them. I have all your *Eating Better Cookbooks* and they are all I ever use. My family loves your recipes and they are healthy and taste great! I sent the books to show you how wonderful and flavorful your recipes are [in comparison,] as well as hassle-free to make. I don't need a special diet plan. I'm losing weight on the *Eating Better* plan—15 lbs. so far!"

Do You Really Need to Lose Weight?

Perhaps the desire to lose weight needs reevaluation. Statistically, persons who are 20% or more overweight have more diabetes, heart disease, and many other health problems. For persons who are only five to ten pounds overweight, the purpose for losing weight may be primarily cosmetic. Be serious about answering this question: "Is God interested in my losing weight or am I merely listening to the voice of my cultural value system?" It may be better not to be concerned about that extra five or ten pounds because once on the dieting merry-go-round it is very difficult to get off, and a worse weight problem may be the unhappy result. Sue tells how she made this mistake while pregnant with her first child. She was so worried about gaining more than the allotted 20 pounds that she began to count calories and plunged herself into years of merry-go-round counting and yo-yo weight fluctuations. Only the *Eating Better Lifestyle*, high in dietary fiber and low in fat, rescued her and stabilized her weight.

What About Compulsive Eating?

The *Eating Better Lifestyle* does not cure compulsive eating behavior. It may assist to curb behavior that has a physiological basis such as an addiction to sugar, but behavior rooted in emotional needs may require special counseling. There are several Christian ministries from which you can get additional support. The restraint of sensual indulgences (Colossians 2:23) can only come by way of an inner work of the Holy Spirit.

Am I a Victim of "Fat Genes"?

Some despairing hearts cry, "All I have to do is look at food and I gain weight!" Why is that? The answer may partly lie in the "fat gene" theory. It may be possible to inherit a physical tendency to produce more, rather than less, fat cells. The clue to such a condition is fat relatives.

Yet many cannot lay claim to a fat family. They also battle with weight because the refined American Diet has contributed to a fat-producing metabolism. Metabolism determines how the body burns calories. Aerobic exercise can alter body metabolism. Exercise contributes to both weight control and total health. It is nutrition's twin.

For further reading we recommend *Beyond Diet* by Martin Katahn, Ph.D. Katahn's two basic rules for weight control are in harmony with the *Eating Better Lifestyle:* 1) Avoid low-calorie diets; and 2) Adopt a high-fiber, low-fat diet. The trend for effective weight loss in the '90s based on extensive research is low-fat eating, not low-calorie eating. Some say that if the fat intake is controlled, the amount of other foods, especially carbohydrates, may be eaten freely without reference to calories. This is particularly true when a low-fat plan is combined with satiating complex carbohydrates that are high in dietary fiber.

While the *Eating Better Lifestyle* focuses on total health, the exchange values are given for each recipe to facilitate their use with diet programs that utilize the exchange system, such as Weight Watchers and 3-D. Following a well-known diet program on the exchange system, Chris remarked, "I'm following this exchange system program substituting your recipes (they're so much tastier and healthier) and I've lost 15 lbs." The exchange system for weight control can be used with *Eating Better Lifestyle* recipes and menus, independently of other programs, by using the plan outlined in **Main Dishes** (see p. 384).

The spiritual discipline of prayer and fasting is also invaluable to weight management. Its purpose is not to "go without calories" in order to lose weight, but to receive spiritual strength, break food cravings and bad habits that mitigate against weight management, and cleanse the body of toxins that interfere (see chapter 45).

If You're Sick 'n Tired
of Being Fat

If you're sick 'n tired of being fat,
  a whole foods diet is where it's at!
Low fat and high fiber, too—
You have everything to gain but weight, in view.

High-fiber calories pass on through
  while many a fat one becomes part of you!
Whole foods chewing takes longer in time;
  you'll find their calories more satisfying.

While refined carbohydrates are a pasty mess
  creating addictions that do not bless,
Succulent fruits and vegetables many
  add vitamins, minerals, and pure water plenty.
These you need to regulate
  all the processes of body
  to properly use what you ate.

More nutrients will more energy devise
  and you'll feel more like exercise.
You'll do more work, and get more done.
Your metabolism will pick up and begin to run.

Give yourself time—this is a slower way,
  but it will last for many a long day.
God looks on the heart,
  not on external appearance.
Thus seek total inner health with
  prayer and perseverance.

—Sue Gregg

30

Exercise: Nutrition's Twin

———— ♥ ————

Do you not know that in a race all the runners run, but only one gets the prize? Run in such a way as to get the prize.

1 Corinthians 9:24

———— ♥ ————

Gone are the days of necessary walking, climbing, running, and sweating to do our daily work! In twentieth-century America we have a unique situation in the history of mankind that conspires against healthy bodies at normal weights—a high-fat, low-fiber diet inadequate in vitamins and minerals plus sedentary lifestyles. Yet our best hope for utilizing most effectively the good food we eat for the total health needs of our bodies is aerobic exercise. Since our work does not provide it, we must create it for ourselves. In general, Christians have recognized and understood the value of exercise for health much better than the nutritional value of whole foods. The result is that we have ample exercise resources available to us through

Christian ministries. Therefore, we will address this need only briefly.

What is aerobic exercise? Simply, it is exercise that increases the oxygen supply in the body and increases the rate of body metabolism. This is valuable to health in many ways. Benefits, most of them interrelated, may include:

> Improved blood cholesterol level
> Normalized blood pressure
> Stabilizing of emotions—lowered
>   depression, anxiety, tension
> Increased physical energy and vitality
> Increased alertness
> Improved elimination
> Detoxification through removal of toxic
>   wastes from body cells
> Healthier cardiovascular system—heart,
>   lungs, etc.
> Improved utilization of food nutrients
> More effective weight loss and maintenance
>   control of weight

Find the type of aerobic exercise that best suits your own circumstances and interests. There are plenty of ways to do it. Check church and community resources for group activity. For exercise at home there are excellent music and videotapes available. Exercise with a friend who lives nearby. It is a great way to maintain mutual accountability and enjoy a conversation break in a busy day.

Emilie walks at least two miles a day, six days a week. She uses the time to pray. Sometimes she sings and just enjoys the beauty around her. The time passes very quickly and she's doing two things at one time. Occasionally she will invite a friend to walk with her just to enjoy each other's fellowship. It takes her 30 minutes to walk two miles. The benefits are great. Good exercise gets her heart rate up, gives her a sense of well-being, and releases stress.

Brisk walking is usually the easiest and most available exercise for everyone, and it is safer for women than jogging. A brisk walk is between 3½ and 4 miles per hour. Buy an inexpensive stopwatch to time your distance. Walking costs no money and often provides a sunshine treat at the same time. In city areas many indoor shopping malls and health clubs have distances marked off for walkers and provide the safety of on-duty security. On rainy days use a cassette or video exercise tape indoors for variety. *Beyond Diet* (see Recommended Reading, p. 379) explains thoroughly how aerobic exercise will alter body metabolism. Author Martin Katahn explains that whole-body activities using the large leg muscles and buttocks to propel your body through space gives the most return for your time and effort. He lists walking and rebounding (jumping on a "minitrampoline") as the best whole-body exercise.[1] Although Sue walks daily with husband, Rich, she prefers a combination of rebounding and exercising to Stormie Omartian's *First Steps* video to walking for aerobic workouts. To each his own. Emilie's Bob finds gardening the most satisfying exercise.

If you are overweight, adopting the *Eating Better Lifestyle* will probably not help you to lose weight on a permanent basis without a regular discipline of aerobic exercise. Make three 20-minute sessions of aerobic exercise your minimum goal each week on alternating days. Incidentally, aerobics is not just for the overweight person. Everyone needs it!

31

Drink Your Way to Health

———— ♥ ————

Everyone who drinks this water will be thirsty again,
but whoever drinks the water I give him will never
thirst. Indeed, the water I give him will become a
spring of water welling up to eternal life.

John 4:13,14

———— ♥ ————

merica loves to drink everything but water—soda
pop, fruit drinks, fruit juices, alcoholic beverages,
coffee, and tea. We guzzle 50 million cans of Coke and 200
million cups of coffee daily. How can plain water possibly
compete?

Water Works!

Approximately three quarts of water are lost from the
human body daily through the kidneys, lungs, and skin. It
must be replaced continually to effectively perform the
work of nutrient transport and elimination of wastes. Two-
thirds water by weight, the body thirsts for nontoxic, clean
water—an increasingly scarce commodity. Agricultural

and industrial wastes have polluted many public water sources. Chlorine, added to kill bacteria, is a health hazard itself. Sodium fluoride, added to protect our teeth from decay, may also be detrimental to health.

What Kind of Water Is Best?

Fresh fruits and vegetables supply part of our water requirement. The water in fresh produce is the purest kind. We can heartily thank our Lord for it. Where, however, is our best source of drinking water?

First, find out the quality of your tap water. Locate a water laboratory that will give you a chemical analysis. Check the yellow pages under "Laboratories—Analytical." An EPA-certified lab has been inspected by the EPA and checked for testing accuracy. If the report lists any of the following chemicals, especially at toxic levels, you should consider an alternative drinking water source: chlorine, sodium fluoride, nitrites, arsenic, barium, cadmium, lead, silver, cyanide, coliform bacteria, or selenium. What alternative sources are best?

Alternatives to tap water include bottled spring water, distilled water, filters on faucets, reverse osmosis, and so on. The options are many and varied. It is often difficult to assess which is most economical, safest, and most effective. We are most familiar with distilled and bottled spring water. Some nutritionists suggest that distilled water leaches minerals from the body over a prolonged period of time. Bill Frisby, however, in *God's HMO* (see Recommended Reading, p. 379) explains that distilled water will not leach out the important cellular minerals because they are strongly bonded to carbon. It will only remove the unwanted mineral deposits as part of the detoxification process.[1] On the other hand, death rates are statistically lower in hard-water areas. The lower death rate is attributed to the higher mineral content in hard water. Yet there can be harmful substances in the hard water, as well. Rich and Sue Gregg decided many years ago to use distilled water, adding mineral seawater purchased from the health-food store to provide any minerals they might have possibly needed. With more information assuring them that distilled water does not leach important minerals from the body, they discontinued this practice. However, if you wish to add a mineral seawater to distilled water, add one to two tablespoons per five gallons water. Purchase only steam-distilled water and not water distilled by deionization. Your tap water may also be distilled with a home distiller. However, after trying a home distilling method, we found home delivery of bottled steamed distilled water much simpler.

If you choose spring water, it is wise to have a chemical analysis of it just as you would your tap water. If you have a water softening system in your home, using it for cooking and drinking is unwise.

The cost of any pure water source is more economical than the American Diet drinking budget!

Should You Drink Water with Meals?

Many health-food enthusiasts tell us not to drink water with meals because it dilutes the digestive juices in the stomach needed to digest food properly. Yet telling most Americans not to drink anything with meals is like telling a man dying of thirst in the hot desert to leave his water flask unopened! So let's be realistic about it. If you want something to drink with the meal, water is to be preferred over soda pop, fruit drinks and juices, and coffee. Keep the risk of diluting digestive juices in mind, however. Sip it a little at a time instead of gulping it or sloshing down food with it. You will discover quickly that the *Eating Better Lifestyle*, which includes lots of fresh fruits and vegetables, will not create as much thirst as meals high in meats and salt. Try drinking water without ice cubes. The body seems to prefer temperatures that are not extreme. Enjoy a refreshing slice of lemon in your water. Lemon will help to purify the water.

How Much Should You Drink Between Meals?

Few people drink more water than they need. Usually we must tell ourselves that we need it. If you are a non-water-drinker, drink one more glass of water a day than you now drink for a week. Increase it by an additional glass per day each week until you are up to one-third your weight in ounces of water. For example, if you weigh 120 lbs., divide 120 by 3 which equals 40, and drink 40 oz. water a day (that's five 8 oz. glasses). Measure out the water quota for the day in the morning. If you need a reminder to drink up, set a timer for every half-hour or hour and drink 4 to 8 oz. each time. Allow 30 minutes between a drink of water and the beginning and end of mealtimes. Drink room temperature water. It goes down better than cold water.

If you do not care for the taste of your water, it may be the combination of chemicals and minerals in the tap water, or even in the bottled water. Many people purchase a particular bottled water just for better taste—a good plan if it encourages you to drink more! Sue, for example, has come to love the "untaste" of distilled water.

I Must Have My Morning Cup of Coffee!

That morning cup just gives me the get-up-and-go, the energy, the alertness, and the vigor to start my day! Do I have to give it up?

Nutritionally, coffee has nothing to offer. It stirs up the nervous system, but does not build strength. Research suggests a mixture of blessings and curses from coffee drinking. Reactions appear to be highly individual. Most troubles begin after the third cup, or about 200 milligrams of caffeine consumed within a 24-hour period. The following reactions are good reasons for quitting or cutting back on the caffeine habit: heartburn or gastrointestinal discomfort, irregular or increased heartbeat, high blood pressure, insomnia, irritability, a need to increase the amount in order to experience a sense of well-being, withdrawal symptoms such as headache and excessive fatigue or depression, frequency of urination, and diarrhea. Those who have ulcers, fibrocystic breast disease, high blood cholesterol, or are pregnant would be wise not to drink coffee. It also consumes thiamine (B_1) and iron, which can aggravate an anemic condition, and leaches calcium out of the body—a nutrient few people can afford to be robbed of.

Some of coffee's effects are related to ingredients other than caffeine. For example, the oil caffeol can irritate the stomach lining, and chlorgenic acid can burn up some of the body's thiamine and iron stores. Decaffeinated coffee also contains these ingredients. Therefore, it may not be the best coffee replacement. Although some people worry about the chemical used to decaffeinate coffee, it generally does not get into the coffee. An alternative, however, is Swiss or water-processed coffee (available at health-food stores if not in the supermarket).

The caffeine habit can be broken gradually or cold turkey. Expect withdrawal symptoms with the cold-turkey method. These probably won't last more than a day or two. Start diluting each cup with a little water, increasing it to half a cup. Low-fat or nonfat milk added to coffee will weaken its acidy abrasiveness in the stomach. Cremora or Coffee-mate contain sugar and are not good substitutes for real milk. Reduce or omit sugar or substitute half as much granulated fructose. Gradually move on to black tea and finally to herb teas. A short fast of up to three days can often break the craving for caffeine.

Take Time for Tea

Although black tea also contains caffeine, it has some advantages. Black tea can help alleviate mild headache, depression, and fatigue without as many risks as coffee. For example, black tea has not been found to raise blood cholesterol. Some of the properties in black tea can actually be beneficial according to "A Drink The Day After," *American*

Health Magazine, April 1984: Polyphenols in tea work with vitamin C to strengthen blood vessel walls. Tea can inhibit growth of decay-causing bacteria in dental plaque, helps to fight colds, helps to minimize effects of radiation, and contains zinc, manganese, and potassium. It can reduce iron absorption, however. This is not a license to drink ten cups a day! But it is an improvement over coffee. Tea contains one-and-a-half to two grains of caffeine per cup as compared with two to four grains in a cup of coffee, depending on how strong each is brewed.

Herb teas are safe and enjoyable in moderation. Each herb contains different medicinal properties. Some of them, if consumed to excess, can cause reactions. It is best not to drink many cups of the same kind. Teas made from peppermint, spearmint, and rose hips are good. The many supermarket blends are fine in moderation (two or three cups a day). Peppermint can soothe mild stomach discomfort, and chamomile can be very soothing for mild headaches.

To make teas, pour boiling water over a tea bag or one teaspoon loose tea and let it steep for five minutes. Remove the tea bag or loose tea before you drink it. Iced herb tea can be delightful, too. To make sun tea, put two tea bags per quart of water in a covered glass jar and set it outdoors in the sun for a few hours.

Juice It!

"We've quit the Kool-Aid, but we still get confused between juice drinks and juice. What's the difference?" Juice drinks are a blend of water, sugar, and perhaps 10% real juice. Fruit juices are all real juice, either unsweetened or sweetened. These all keep company on the same shelf in the supermarket. Read labels carefully to select the real and unsweetened juices. Bottled juices are to be preferred over canned. Unsweetened frozen juice concentrates, also occupying cozy quarters with the sweetened variety, are also good choices.

Even real juices are refined foods because they have been extracted from the whole fruits. This removes the dietary fiber and concentrates the sugar, even if it is natural. That doesn't mean to quit drinking real fruit juice. It is an improvement over soda pop and fruit drinks, but juice can't match the value of fresh fruit. Dilute fruit juice 50-50 with water to cut the sugar concentration and halve the price!

Fresh fruit and vegetable juices are in a class by themselves. None of the enzymes or other nutrient values have been destroyed by canning. Fresh juices can be very beneficial in cleansing the system during a short fast of up to three days. Sue's favorite fresh juice combinations are available in **Breakfasts** (see p. 384). A delightful book on juicing with great recipes is *The Juiceman's Power of Juicing* by Jay Kordich, available at health-food stores and most bookstores.

What about the fiber lost in juicing? Are you going to sit down to a pound of carrots if you don't juice them? You'll get plenty of *Eating Better Lifestyle* fiber, juice or no juice. So take advantage of this wonder-working powerhouse of nutrients and cleansing. Drink an 8-oz. glass daily, or periodically enjoy a three-day fast with fresh juices!

32

Mind, Mood, and Food

—————— ♥ ——————

Love the Lord your God with all your heart and with all
your soul and with all your mind.

Matthew 22:37

—————— ♥ ——————

"After Thanksgiving dinner I felt like taking a l-o-n-g winter's nap!" We can say amen to that! The effects of nutrients on the brain is a fascinating new field of research and experimentation. Judith J. Wurtman, Ph.D., has published an entire book on the subject: *Managing Your Mind and Mood Through Food* (Rawson Associates, New York, 1986). Nutrients do indeed affect mental clarity, emotions, and behavior. For example, starchy carbohydrates eaten alone will stimulate the release of serotonin, a neurotransmitter in the brain. Serotonin produces calmness and sleepiness. In contrast, protein suppresses the serotonin and wakes you up! Nonstarchy carbohydrates such as leafy greens, broccoli, and brightly colored fresh fruits don't affect the level of serotonin either way. Wurtman suggests that you eat protein with starchy carbohydrates to stay awake and alert. Eating food low in fat and not overeating is also important for a clear mind. That means save the spaghetti for dinner so you can relax afterward and eat the tuna and lettuce on rye for lunch for a more mentally alert afternoon. Wurtman explains that this is the general pattern, but there are individual exceptions.

Does Food Affect Criminal Behavior?

Alexander Schauss, director of the American Institute for Biosocial Research and author of *Diet, Crime, and Delinquency*, has been instrumental in changing the nutritional quality of foods offered to prison inmates. The rates of recidivism (return to crime) have dropped significantly among juvenile delinquents and criminals who have been given better food. Says Bernard Fensterwald, III, NNFA Legislative Counsel: "Massive consumption of refined carbohydrates and other questionable substances by prison inmates causes severe behavior problems. Undeniably, they are more aggressive—which leads to more assaults, homosexual rapes and the like. At a minimum, they are continually disoriented and often act irrationally. Their ability to concentrate is impaired, and this lessens the prison's rehabilitation effort."[1]

Nutritional Therapy?

Research into the therapeutic use of food nutrients is demonstrating their value to health far beyond what we have traditionally understood. Nutrients in a variety of research projects have helped persons who are mentally retarded, mentally ill, emotionally disturbed, autistic, senile, delinquent, criminal, and slow learners. Almost all of the nutrients have been used in megadoses in varying ways and combinations, most notably the B-vitamins. Orthomolecular research is a branch entirely devoted to the nutritional approach to mental problems. See Recommended Reading, p. 380 under "Foods for Healing" for resource books that suggest therapeutic uses of vitamins and minerals plus other food supplements for specific health conditions.

Does Nutrition Keep a Mind Healthy?

The effect of nutrition on mental behavior is currently viewed with skepticism by conservative scientists and researchers. For example, the value of the Feingold diet and the value of reducing refined sugar to fight hyperactivity in children have both been recently challenged. Yet the early evidence that nutrients are vital to mental health and behavior is promising.

We have introduced this aspect of nutrition to further inspire you to develop the *Eating Better Lifestyle*. If persons with the mental afflictions we have mentioned are being helped by nutritional therapy, we wonder how many of these afflictions could be minimized or prevented by the *Eating Better Lifestyle*. It is becoming clearer that our minds and emotions depend upon physiological and chemical reactions in our bodies. "Love the Lord your God with all your . . . mind" (Matthew 22:37) suggests that doing those things which enhance our potential to respond to God's Word and to the indwelling Holy Spirit is worthy of our attention.

33

But I Love My Chocolate!

———— ♥ ————

"Everything is permissible for me"—but not everything is beneficial. *"Everything is permissible for me"*—
but I will not be mastered by anything.

1 Corinthians 6:12

———— ♥ ————

The hardest things to give up are those that we love!
We can find all sorts of rationalizations for hanging
on to them. Will it help a little if we say that you can "have
your chocolate cake and eat it, too"? That's right! The white
flour and the white sugar may be worse than the chocolate
in it. You can make chocolate cake with whole-wheat flour
and honey. In fact, in home baking you can use chocolate in
any recipe along with other ingredients that are more nutritious. But if you want to buy commercial sweets with
chocolate, you are in trouble! Chocolate keeps company
with nutritionally unsavory ingredients! So if you love

chocolate candies and other commercial chocolate creations, we suggest that you set a goal to prepare more wholesome homemade goodies—even if they do contain chocolate.

In spite of your chocolate love, we want to introduce the benefits of carob. Carob does not aggravate skin problems, contribute to digestive troubles, or cause allergic reactions as chocolate frequently does. Chocolate is especially high on the list of allergens, while practically no one reacts to carob.

Carob belongs to the legume family of beans and peas such as lentils and split peas. Therefore, it shares similar nutritional benefits. Carob is an excellent source of calcium, potassium, pectin, and bowel-regulating dietary fiber, and contains iron, vitamin A, and vitamins B_1 and B_3. It does not contain the oxalic acid of chocolate that could interfere with calcium absorption and is not high in the stimulant theobromine. Unlike chocolate, it is virtually fat- and caffeine-free. Carob has some of its own natural sweetness, while chocolate is bitter. Therefore carob requires a little less additional sweetening in recipes.

Note how 3 tablespoons of carob powder compare with their equivalent of 1 oz. of chocolate:

	1 oz. Chocolate*	3 tbsp. Carob
Calories	185	47
Fat	15.8 grams (142.0 calories)	0.33 grams (3.0 calories)
Calcium	20 mg.	90 mg.
Theobromine	1047 mg.	0.4 mg.

*Hershey's Baking Chocolate

Chocolate is not totally devoid of nutrients. It does contain vitamin A, B-vitamins, and also more iron and potassium than carob.

What about the flavor of carob? We won't pretend that carob tastes just like chocolate. It doesn't—especially not to chocolate lovers! Rich, Sue's husband, as a chocolate lover, was not interested in the flavor of carob during the first year of transition to the *Eating Better Lifestyle*. Sue's daughter Sharon still does not care for carob. Yet her home-baked creations that include chocolate also include whole-wheat flour, honey, and other ingredients nutritionally superior to commercial goodies. A halfway measure is a blend of half carob and half chocolate.

Carob is easy to substitute in any recipe. Mix 2 tablespoons hot water with 3 tablespoons carob powder to replace each 1 oz. square of unsweetened chocolate. If cocoa powder is added to the dry ingredients, substitute the same amount of carob powder. Buy roasted carob powder in either the supermarket or the health-food store.

In your favorite chocolate cake recipe, substitute whole-wheat pastry flour for half or more of the white flour. Use half as much honey as sugar. If you want to use chocolate, WonderSlim Pure Low-Fat Cocoa Powder may be purchased in health-food stores and even in some supermarkets. WonderSlim contains no fat and is 99.7% caffeine free. If you are not satisfied with the results, it may be better to start with new recipes already adapted to more nutritious ingredients, such as those in *Eating Better Desserts* (see p. 384).

34

Alterations for Allergies

———— ♥ ————

There is . . . a time to search and a time to give up, a
time to keep and a time to throw away. . . .

Ecclesiastes 3:1,6

———— ♥ ————

*T*he symptoms of allergies or food sensitivities are
often confused with symptoms of other health conditions. Yet many persons who have detected offending
foods and removed them from their diet or limited their use
have found relief from a wide variety of symptoms: tired-
ness, lack of energy, mental confusion or fogginess, depression, crying spells, headaches, irritability, nasal drip,
mucus in the system, rashes, hives, and a host of other
problems.

Before embarking on a detective hunt for food allergies,
be aware of other possible causes of symptoms: a generally
nutrient-poor diet (see p. 86); not enough exercise, rest,
sunshine, fresh air, or drinking water; poor food combinations; the need for vitamin-mineral supplementation;

sensitivities to nonfood items in the environment; an unre-solved relationship or emotions; or lack of peace with God through Christ.*

How to Find a Food Allergy

A health-care professional may suggest allergy tests. These can be expensive and are not always accurate. Envi-ronmental allergens are easier to test than foods. A do-it-yourself elimination diet is less expensive and can be more accurate. The *Do-It-Yourself Allergy Analysis Handbook* by Henderson and Ludeman (see Recommended Reading, p. 379) outlines professional testing methods as well as how to use the elimination diet method. You will find much detailed help in this reference book.

Common food allergens are milk, wheat, eggs, corn, potatoes, tomatoes, citrus fruits, carrots, chicken, beef, peanuts, apples, oats, green beans, soy, and yeast. The first four are the leading allergens in America. Often a problem food is one to which you are addicted. When using a do-it-yourself method, start with the leading food allergens that you eat most often, then move on to the others. It would be wise to first begin with a fast for a few days to cleanse the system and to prepare spiritually. Do-it-yourself detective work will require perseverance. Before fasting, however, be sure to read chapter 45 on prayer and fasting and check the Recommended Reading on pp. 379-80, especially if fast-ing is new to you.

By all means do not embark on a do-it-yourself program without the above-mentioned resource book. Read it prayer-fully before choosing a testing method.

Coping with a Food Allergy

If you are sensitive to many foods, your condition is not necessarily irreversible. Some foods you may never be able

---

* See *Greater Health God's Way* by Stormie Omartian.

to include. Others you may be able to begin to enjoy with care. Though you have a milk allergy, you may be able to tolerate milk in cultured form. Children often outgrow food allergies.

Ingredient Alternatives

The four leading allergens—milk and milk products, wheat, eggs, and corn—are used in many different recipes and packaged foods. Our recipes in the *Eating Better Cookbooks* (see pp. 383-84) include ingredient alternatives for these foods. For wheat there are tasty recipes using other whole grains. Spelt and Kamut, whole grains recently available in America, can be used successfully in yeast breads and other recipes. While spelt and Kamut are wheat, many persons allergic to the common varieties of wheat can tolerate them. Brown rice and barley work well in cookies, cakes, and pie crusts in place of wheat. These alternatives are presented in *Eating Better Desserts*. Our muffins, pancakes, and waffles also offer ample grain alternatives to wheat. Many recipes are included in *Eating Better Breakfasts* and *Soups & Muffins*.

While wheat is a leading allergen, gluten intolerance—a rather severe reaction to gluten in grains—is not so common, but possible. *Good Food, Gluten Free* by Hilda Cherry Hills (Keats Publishing, Inc., New Canaan, Connecticut, 1976), is a good resource to help in coping with gluten intolerance.

Corn allergy need not be an obstacle in home cooking. Low-sodium baking powder does not contain corn. You can use arrowroot powder in place of cornstarch. Arrowroot and low-sodium baking powder are available at health-food stores. Yeast can also contain corn, but *Red Star* brand does not. If allergic to yeast, prepare quick bread recipes such as whole-grain muffins, cornbread, and popovers instead. Sourdough and sprouted breads digest more easily. You may be able to tolerate these. Some persons allergic to wheat can tolerate wheat in the sprouted form. Nondairy and dairy alternatives to use in place of sweet milk are listed in chapter 24, pp. 129, 132. In all baking and milk-based soups, a tasty soy milk is most versatile (such as Better Than Milk brand). In soups you can also use vegetable, beef, or chicken stock, thickened with potatoes in place of milk. Use the blender to make creamy non-milk soups.

For egg alternatives, see pp. 121-22.

35

Ode to Pesky Preservatives and Poisonous Pesticides

———— ♥ ————

Spray the crops to grow more than we need;
refine them before the people we feed.
Dress them up with color and taste;
of good whole food, what a waste!

How much preservative I can't tell.
But it is added to everything
so that it might sell.
If you want food, pesticide free,
you can grow your own
for a very small fee.

Some places you can buy it
organ-i-cal-ly.
Speak to the farmer,
speak to the grocer,
speak to the health-food store owner.
You'll find a supply, by and by,
if you are but willing to try.
Watch at the supermarket—
some might be sold there.

Organic foods may cost a bit more
when we buy them from the store;
but of purer food we'll not be poor.

And whatever those thousands of additives be,
of them all we can be free.
Just read those labels
and buy food that is whole
and be healthier
in spirit, body, and soul!

—*Sue Greg*

Organically Grown

Organic food is generally defined as grown without the use of pesticides and commercial fertilizers. There are various programs that set standards for certification of products. For example, two independent certification companies that follow internationally recognized standards for the organic food industry are FVO (Farm Verified Organic) and OCIA (Organic Crop Improvement Association). It is important that so-called "organic" foods be certified by an independent company with high standards. If food is labeled organic, request certification documentation by independent sources such as FVO or OCIA. Insufficient legal documentation does not mean that it is not organic. It means you must rely on the word of the farmer, wholesaler, and retailer.

"Poly-WHAT?"

If EDTA, poly-something, disodium-whatever, and mono- and di-what-have-you are a foreign language, you need Ruth Winter's *Consumer's Dictionary of Food Additives* (see Recommended Reading, p. 379). When you are tempted to buy a "chemical conglomerate" that is supposed to represent real food, or find a "unfood item" in an ingredients label, look the additives up in the *Consumer's Dictionary*. It will be invaluable for making wise packaged food choices!

Safe Food by Jacobson, Lefferts, and Garland (see p. 380) lists the top ten additives to avoid, with explanations:

Acesulfame K, a sugar substitute (commercially sold as Sunette or Sweet One),

Artificial colorings

Aspartame (commercially sold as NutraSweet and Equal)

BHA

BHT

Caffeine (besides being natural to coffee, tea, and cocoa, it is added to soft drinks)

MSG (monosodium glutamate)

Nitrite and nitrate

Saccharin

Sulfites

36

Questions Often Asked

———— ♥ ————

*A man finds joy in giving an apt reply—and how good
is a timely word!*

Proverbs 15:23

———— ♥ ————

Are you nutritionists?

No. Our focus is on homemaking. We do this by teaching principles of healthful living and how to apply them in the home to kitchen and household organization, shopping, menu planning, and food preparation. As such we are the women of Titus 2:4,5 who ". . . train the younger women to love their husbands and children, to be self-controlled and pure, to be busy at home, to be kind. . . ."

The title of "nutritionist" usually designates a person who assists those with specific health problems to set up individualized diet programs. Nutritionists frequently use various kinds of tests to determine an individual's dietary needs. They often work with a medical doctor, especially one who focuses on preventive care. The doctor will provide the diagnosis and the nutritionist then provides the diet program. Our menus and recipes serve as resources for the nutritionist.

Do you have a diet for diabetics?

The *Eating Better Lifestyle* is not a therapeutic diet for any disease or health condition. Its purpose is preventive family health care. It is, however, adaptable to therapeutic diets. For example, all of our recipes include exchange values comparable to the exchange system recommended by the American Diabetes Association. The *Eating Better Lifestyle* is also a high-fiber lifestyle—important for diabetics. Our sugar alternatives for refined sugar are also helpful.

Therapeutic diets are designed with the help of a health professional such as a preventive care medical doctor or nutrition consultant. A worthwhile reference for the home library is *A Prescription for Nutritional Healing: A Practical A–Z Reference*, by James F. Balch, M.D., and Phyllis Balch, C.N.C., available at health-food stores.

Is fasting safe and should I do it? Is it a good way to lose weight?

Fasting is safe if done properly and has many benefits. It can be valuable in gaining control over a weight problem, but we do not recommend it as a primary means for losing weight. See "Why Low-Calorie Diets Don't Work," (pp. 159-60) and "Prayer and Fasting" (chapter 45). Anorexia is an extreme form of fasting to prevent weight gain.

Are herb teas a good substitute for caffeinated beverages such as coffee, black tea, or cola drinks?

Yes. (See pp. 173-74.)

If I quit using iodized table salt, will I get enough iodine?

This question belies the source of most Americans' nutritional education—advertising. Few are worried, for example, about getting enough magnesium. We worry about iodine, however, because the label on the iodized salt box states that "iodine is an essential nutrient." Table salt was iodized originally to compensate for iodine deficiency of the soil in the Great Lakes region. The soil is not iodine deficient everywhere. Seafoods, both plant and animal, contain iodine. Kelp is one of the richest sources and some people choose to use it in place of salt in cooking. It is an excellent choice. If you do not care for the taste, it can be added to the diet in tablet form. Sea salt that has not been kiln dried does not contain the RDA of iodine, although it contains traces. Seawater that might be added to distilled water (p. 170) contains iodine. According to *Safe Food* by Jacobson, Lefferts, and Garland, too much iodine in the diet is now possible due to iodized salt added to many packaged foods and foods exposed to iodine used as an antiseptic. Our choice of salt is *RealSalt*, an unrefined mined salt from Utah, available in many health-food stores and by mail order (see p. 304).

What do you think of NutraSweet?

We suggest caution in its use. (See p. 150.)

What do you think about microwave ovens? Do you have recipes for the microwave?

Admittedly, the microwave oven is the "miracle" appliance of our time for busy people who forget to thaw the meat in the refrigerator and for those who can't be bothered with meal preparation until ten minutes before the meal! The *Eating Better Lifestyle* encourages families to do better than this. We have collected information about microwave cooking in the last couple of years that suggests much caution in the use of the microwave oven. Preliminary research studies suggest that microwave cooking may be cause for concern in at least three areas: 1) possible cancer-causing and cholesterol-raising effects, 2) negative effects on the nutritive value of foods, and 3) possible effects of direct microwave oven radiation emissions. Research studies have established that heating a baby's bottle of milk in the microwave changes the quality of the milk protein, making it unfit for baby's health. If microwaving does this to baby's milk, what about other food protein? Clearly, more research is needed, as this goes contrary to all we've heard about the microwave preserving nutrients in foods!

In the meantime, while we do not have recipes for the microwave, we have incorporated certain steps of food preparation using the microwave in the *Eating Better Cookbooks*—generally as an option to standard cooking. This is minimal, however, and standard cooking directions are provided as well.

Sue originally purchased a microwave oven to thaw and reheat freezer casseroles. She now uses it primarily as a very accurate timer for whatever's cooking in her gas oven—an expensive timer! Oh yes! She does resort to thawing the meat in the microwave occasionally—on defrost—like when her husband, Rich, brought home the ground turkey for hamburgers last week, ten minutes before the meal—frozen solid.

I have heard that honey has more calories than sugar and causes tooth decay. Is this true?

Honey has slightly more calories than sugar. One tablespoon of honey has 64 calories compared to one tablespoon of sugar's 50 calories, but such a comparison is not practically meaningful since honey is twice as sweet. One-and-a-half teaspoons of honey will sweeten as well as one tablespoon of sugar, so in reality you consume fewer calories.

As for tooth decay, it would be more accurate to say, "Excess honey can cause tooth decay." When we teach about the value of using honey in place of white refined sugar, we are not suggesting excessive use of honey. We do not suggest that a person substitute an average intake of 120 pounds of sugar, for example, with 120 pounds of honey, or even 60 pounds of honey. We suggest using it in quite small amounts. We ought to brush our teeth and teach our children to brush their teeth shortly after eating anything containing sugar other than that in fresh fruits.

What do you think of food combining?

Those who advocate food-combining rules (p. 102) try to give what they believe is a scientific basis for the practice. But we are not fully satisfied with the explanation. Ruth Bircher in *Eating Your Way to Health* presents the position of the Bircher-Benner Clinic in Zurich, Switzerland: "We have tried to study this problem in detail but neither have we found sufficient facts which could be considered scientifically conclusive, nor have we found in our own clinical experience sufficient reasons for giving such general rules for the feeding of healthy people or invalids. Therefore, we do not feel justified in renouncing in principle all those natural, time-honored and valuable tasty combinations of healthy foods, such as 'potatoes and cream cheese', 'milk and cereals', 'apples and bread', which are all forbidden by these schools of thought. Such combinations are found particularly in the diets of the healthiest people in food geography or history. . . . The incompatibility of certain foods is, in our opinion, something which has to be considered very carefully with each individual invalid by examining his reactions in each particular case. But it is really concerned with the invalid diet of the individual patient, not with the general teaching of dietetics."[1]

There are persons, however, who have been helped by adopting a diet based on food-combining guidelines. They have experienced more energy, better digestion, and help with weight loss and control. It is worthy of individual consideration, but we do not advocate it as a general pattern essential to the *Eating Better Lifestyle*. Many of our recipes are properly food combined or adaptable to proper food combining for those who want to follow that pattern. Limited food combining is a very difficult pattern for most

Americans to adopt. Such loved dishes as spaghetti and meat balls, cheese pizza, hamburgers, lasagna, cereal with fruit, eggs and toast, and pancakes with syrup are not allowed on such a diet. The all-American cheese or tuna sandwich is out of the question even if you do use whole wheat bread and cheddar cheese or water-pack unsalted tuna with dark green leafy lettuce and sprouts! We believe it is an unrealistic approach for most Americans. " 'People's food habits change very slowly,' say most anthropologists."[2] We believe the challenges that we have presented for change are more important for most people than food combining.

Should I drink water with meals?

With some caution. (See p. 171.)

Isn't margarine healthier to eat than butter? I thought butter was saturated fat. Aren't there any healthy alternatives?

Butter is saturated fat, but margarine is not a better choice (see pp. 107-08). New substitute and lower-fat products for butter seem to be endless. You can't ask someone else to evaluate each of these products for you, because the parade of new ones never ends! Rather, get the tools you need to evaluate a new product for yourself. Purchase a copy of *A Consumer's Dictionary of Food Additives* by Ruth Winter (see Recommended Reading p. 379). Carry it in your car. It can serve as your "right hand" for evaluating the ingredients in new products. In addition, memorize the list of the top ten additives to avoid (p. 188). Finally, avoid all packaged foods with partially hydrogenated or hydrogenated fat of any type (this will eliminate about half the packaged foods on supermarket shelves).

One possible alternative to butter is nonhydrogenated Spectrum Naturals Spread, made with canola oil. The ingredients label reads: 100% Pure Pressed Canola Oil, Water, Sea Salt, Xanthan and Guar Gum, Soy Protein Isolate,

Annato, Citric Acid, Sorbic Acid at $1/10$ of 1% (anti-mold agent), Natural Butter Flavor (nondairy soy-based), Tumeric. Look each of those up in *A Consumer's Dictionary*, to find out why each ingredient is needed and if it's safe to eat. Then buy a box at the health-food store and see if you like it. In the meantime, try *Butter Spread* (p. 371), our own alternative to butter.

What do you think of salt substitutes?

We don't believe salt substitutes are necessary. Usually the flavor of salt substitutes leaves something to be desired. But do use a quality sea salt. Read chapter 28.

I just love ice cream. Is there anything healthier I can eat that can take its place?

Yes, there are some good frozen yogurts. Ask shops that sell frozen yogurt to show you the ingredients label of their product. Try to avoid refined sugar and a long list of chemicals. With the standardized nutrient data labeling now being required by law on all packaged foods, you can quickly find out the fat content (see chapter 58 on reading labels). Try our recipe for *Frozen Vanilla Yogurt* (p. 370).

I've heard that it is not a good idea to use a lot of oil because it is so high in fat. What about olive oil?

Olive oil is an excellent choice. Balance it with the use of some polyunsaturated oils for the essential fatty acids (see chapter 21).

I am hearing about "irradiated" foods. What are they? Are they safe to buy?

Food irradiation is becoming an important issue. Irradiated food is food treated by radiation to disinfect it, increasing shelf life from days to weeks. It may also destroy insects such as the Mediterranean fruit fly, reduce the need for spraying foods with chemical preservatives after harvesting, reduce the need for nitrates and nitrites in foods, destroy trichinosis organisms in pork, curb salmonella in poultry, and reduce botulism in cured meats. The FDA accepts the relative safety of irradiation and its advantages over whatever low risks there might be.

Irradiated food is not radioactive. But according to *Nutrition Action Healthletter*, "It cannot be stated with certainty that irradiated food is dangerous—or safe."[3] There are several reasons for this uncertainty. Various animal tests show conflicting results. More complete studies are needed. Some nutrient loss may occur at higher doses of irradiation than the FDA is now considering.

Mass irradiation of our food supply may be delayed by the controversy. Foods being considered for irradiation include wheat, fish, poultry, pork, beef, fresh fruits, and fresh vegetables. The current irradiation labeling law permits irradiated foods to be sold without careful labeling. At present, irradiated ingredients can be used in packaged foods and in restaurants without labeling. Labeling should be made clear on all food products so consumers can make informed choices. For more information about the food irradiation issue, contact: Health and Energy Institute, 236 Massachusetts Avenue, N.E., Suite 506, Washington, D.C. 20002, (202) 543-1070; or National Coalition to Stop Food Irradiation, Box 59-0488, San Francisco, CA 94159, (415) 56N-CSFI. An excellent reading resource is *Food Irradiation, Who Wants It?* (see p. 380). Get it at a health-food store.

Is aluminum cookware safe? I have heard that aluminum causes Alzheimer's disease.

Alzheimer's disease has been related in some studies to high aluminum levels, but no conclusions have been reached.

Highly acidic foods such as apples, tomatoes, or recipes

with apple cider vinegar, lemon juice, or other citrus juices are best prepared in non-aluminum cookware and stored in something besides aluminum foil. Other foods, however, probably do not absorb any significant amount of aluminum. Aluminum used in food products may be of greater concern since the concentration is many times higher than what might come from aluminum pots. For most cooking and baking we recommend stainless steel or glass as the safest for health. Ceramic Crockpots are also acceptable. The occasional use of an aluminum pan (to bake a cake, for example), need not be of great concern. Certain bakeware items are hardly available in anything but aluminum, such as angel food cake tube pans and bundt pans. To freeze food in aluminum foil, wrap it first in plastic wrap, then in the foil.

What is the best food for babies?

The best food for a baby is a well-nourished mother and father before conception. If you have not yet begun a family, adopting the *Eating Better lifestyle* for yourself and your spouse is the best foundation. When the baby is born, mother's milk is superb. A baby well-nourished on mother's milk should not need any solid food before six months of age. Solids may be introduced between six and 12 months, but mother's milk is still the main food.

Introduce only one food at a time and watch for any negative reactions before adding a new food. Do not force-feed any food a baby rejects. A baby's digestive system is sensitive and allergies can develop easily. Start grains only after one year. For babies six months or older, table food ground in a baby-food grinder or blender provides better food than jars of commercial baby food.

For more information about feeding babies or small children, see Recommended Reading (p. 379) under Children & Infants, Feeding & Teaching.

What do you think of frozen vegetables? Are they good to eat?

Choose fresh vegetables as much as you can, filling in with frozen vegetables for variety. Frozen vegetables are much to be preferred over canned vegetables, where nutrient loss is greater.

How do home-canned fruits and vegetables fit into the Eating Better Lifestyle? I have a large garden.

By all means preserve excess garden produce! There is a proverb: "Go to the ant, you sluggard; consider its ways and be wise! It has no commander, no overseer or ruler, yet it stores its provisions in summer and gathers its food at harvest" (Proverbs 6:6-8). Fruits can be canned in a honey syrup instead of white sugar. Use half as much honey as you would sugar in a light syrup. Jams can be made with mild-flavored honey or granulated fructose. Recipes for strawberry or apricot preserves, peach or apple butter are available in **Eating Better Lunches & Snacks** (see p. 384 for information).

Choose freezing fresh produce over canning. You might also want to consider a dehydrator as an alternative to canning. Dehydrated fruits and vegetables preserve more nutrients than either freezing or canning.

PART 5

--- ♥ ---

Biblical Perspectives

--- ♥ ---

37

The Value of the Human Body

---- ♥ ----

When I consider your heavens, the work of your fingers, the moon and the stars, which you have set in place, what is man that you are mindful of him, the son of man that you care for him? You made him a little lower than the heavenly beings and crowned him with glory and honor.

Psalm 8:3-5

---- ♥ ----

*O*f all God's creative works, one is very special—man and woman created in His image. The psalmist sang, "For you created my inmost being; you knit me together in my mother's womb. I praise you because I am fearfully and wonderfully made" (Psalm 139:13,14). The human being is awesomely complex.

Yet twentieth-century Christians elevate the value of the spirit over the body almost universally. The body is finite. The spirit is eternal. The result is that Christians consider bodily care less important than spiritual care. John White describes our misunderstanding in *The Masks of Melancholy*: "Most of us possess a muddled mixture of Greek and Hebrew thought which we have inherited in part through Plato, Aristotle, the Gnostics, St. Thomas Aquinas and the philosopher Descartes. We have divided the human being up into a less important physical part (body and brain) and a more important immaterial part (mind and soul)."[1] White's illustration of the interdependence of body and spirit is illuminating: "To compare mind with body is like comparing music with the pianist's fingers. 'What matters is the music!' we cry. Of course. But no fingers, no music. Clumsy fingers, bad music. Weak fingers, feeble music."[2]

Scripture teaches that when someone receives Christ, the Holy Spirit comes to dwell in his/her body. The human spirit does not leave the body to dwell with God. Instead, the Holy Spirit comes to live in the physical body of the new believer (1 Corinthians 6:19).

Another mistake we have made is to view the human body as somehow evil. The apostle Paul said, "I know that nothing good lives in me, that is, in my sinful nature" (Romans 7:18). The King James Version of the Bible uses the word *flesh* instead of *sinful nature*. We have misunderstood *flesh* to mean the physical body—"No good thing dwells in my physical body." This is entirely incorrect! Man's sin nature is the condition of his spirit, not his physical body! The body is subject to sickness, decay, and death not because it is sinful or evil in itself, but because it is a victim of man's sinful nature.

The body, on the other hand, is God's key instrument through which He communicates Himself to the world. It should be self-evident, therefore, that He wills for us to take care of our bodies wisely, conscientiously, and faithfully. It should be no surprise that God has put into nature a complex nutritional fueling system for this purpose.

A wise owner of a new automobile will heed the instructions of the operations and maintenance manual, written by the auto manufacturer to ensure its optimum performance. The car owner will not select the wrong fuel in order to save time, money, or effort. God has also given us an instruction manual for our incredible human body. The first instruction is to understand ourselves as whole persons, not as disembodied spirits. New Age philosophy would like to separate bodies from spirits, but God does not. Even the separation of our bodies from our spirits at death is temporary. On resurrection day, the dead in Christ will be raised to life—new bodies reunited with their spirits. Those alive in Christ will have their decaying living bodies changed to imperishable ones. We will all sit down (in physically imperishable bodies just like Christ's resurrection body in Luke 24:40-43) at the wedding banquet table with the Lamb of God—our Redeemer, Jesus Christ—and dine on food!

Throughout this book we have already made application of God's Word to the subject of food. In the following chapters we want to add a bit more from God's "instruction manual." We cannot exhaust the subject, but want to raise awareness so it will be clear that our foundation for the *Eating Better Lifestyle* is solid biblically. While this may not appear important on the surface, it is vital because we are surrounded by approaches to diet and health that oppose the purpose of the Christian life.

38

God Has a Plan for Health

———— ♥ ————

He forgives all my sins and heals all my diseases, he redeems my life from the pit and crowns me with love and compassion. He satisfies my desires with good things so that my youth is renewed like the eagle's.

from Psalm 103:3-5

———— ♥ ————

The Bible is our most important health manual. Our God is truly our Great Physician. The Old Testament health laws, the restoration of Job to health, the healing ministries of the prophets Elijah and Elisha, our Lord's own healing ministry, and the promise of an eternity without sin and sickness all attest to God's plan for healthful living. "There can be no question that Jesus Christ regarded illness as something to overcome. He did not acquiesce to it. He did not ignore it. He did not content himself with making the best use of it, important as this is when illness is not removed. He coped with illness, and he conquered it. It was his teaching that God wills healing, and he interpreted his healing acts as signs of God's power in the world and of God's ultimate intention to redeem the whole man."[1] When the leper came to Jesus and said, "If you are willing, you can make me clean," Jesus replied, "I am willing. . . . be clean!" (Mark 1:40,41).

Creation is also a witness to God's powerful healing character. His "invisible qualities—his eternal power and divine nature—have been clearly seen, being understood from what has been made, so that men are without excuse" (Romans 1:20). This means that, even without the Bible, man can see the power and holiness of God in nature. "Natural law is God's law, and the more we learn of physiological. . . processes the greater is our awareness of the vast intelligence of the Creator."[2] For example, He has put many mechanisms in our bodies both to protect us from and to fight danger and disease. Pain is a very useful physical response that not only keeps our fingers from getting burned on a hot stove, but also ensures that we will rest during sickness to give the body a better chance to heal. Pain signals that something is wrong so that we will seek a remedy. Sickness is our experience of the body's fight to stay well. Fever, for example, is caused by the war of the white blood cells against infectious bacteria. When a finger is cut or a knee is bruised, the body undertakes an intricate process of healing. Our bodies are designed to continuously operate for health and wellness. We also see that natural things such as food, water, and oxygen keep us alive. We know that the vitamin D from sunshine is needed for strong bones and teeth. Creation cries out with a loud message: "God is willing to heal sickness."

We cannot blame God then for sickness and death. The source of these lies elsewhere. Man subjected himself to sickness and death when Adam and Eve chose to rebel against God's command in the Garden of Eden. We have inherited a sinful nature. Because of our sinful nature we make wrong choices. Much personal suffering (though certainly not all) results from our own wrong choices. For example, the choice to smoke can result in lung cancer, the choice to drink excessively can lead to a diseased liver, the choice to eat refined food can lead to chronic constipation or to colon cancer. Much of our sickness and untimely death is inflicted by choices, including poor lifestyle choices. We are not merely ill-fated victims of such tragedies. Peoples of other cultures who eat native whole foods in their local environment do not suffer these tragedies. What a judgment against us that people who don't know God or His Son, Jesus, reap the benefits of His natural laws better than we do! God has put standards for health into the creation and in His Word. He can expect Christians to heed them.

39

Prevention, Miracle, and Medicine

———— ♥ ————

All healing is of God, whether it occurs through what we call natural law or according to laws which we do not yet know.[1]

———— ♥ ————

For over 100 years Christian medical missions have been operating throughout the world, but the people they serve are just as sick as ever. Medical missionaries are learning what many Americans are learning. Crisis medicine to cure illness does not remove the cause. Medical missions are now taking a close look at what is called primary health care. Primary health care means establishing such things as clean water supplies, adequate food, nutrition, and sanitation. Primary health care is taking advantage of God's preventive measures for good health. It means following His health standards. That is what the *Eating*

Better Lifestyle is all about. It does not provide the sensationalism of a miraculous cure. It means discipline and the challenge of planning health-giving meals. Yet both of these means are equally from God. We should not ignore a healthy lifestyle until we get sick, and then go to the doctor to get "fixed up," or ask God for a miracle cure. God has given us the benefits of all three of these health means— prevention, miracle, and medicine. To carelessly ignore prevention and then cast our sick bodies at the feet of the doctor or at the foot of the cross for a miracle cure is no different than jumping off a building to see if God's holy angels will rescue us in midair (Matthew 4:6,7)!

Primary care for health begins in the home with proper nutrition, wise use of natural remedies, exercise, rest, meaningful work, love and acceptance, companionship, and moral standards. "The importance of home and family in the realm of physical and mental health is very great."[2] Making a plan and working a plan for eating better is essential to the complete primary health care package.

40

Not Health for Health's Sake

---♥---

*The Spirit of the Sovereign LORD is on me, because the
LORD has anointed me to preach good news to the poor.
He has sent me to bind up the brokenhearted, to pro-
claim freedom for the captives and release from dark-
ness for the prisoners, to proclaim the year of the
LORD's favor and the day of vengeance of our God.*
Isaiah 61:1,2

---♥---

*W*hy does our God want us to be in good health? Is it
to make us happy, to make us feel good, to give us
more time to do the things we want to do, to be spared the
pain of sickness, to put off dying as long as possible?

Three examples will help us to put purpose for health
into perspective. These three cases involve the lives of three
persons deeply dedicated to promoting health through better nutrition: Nathan Pritikin, author of *The Pritikin Program*

for Diet and Exercise; Adele Davis, forerunner of the current health-food movement who wrote several books on nutrition such as *Let's Eat Right to Keep Fit*, and *Let's Cook It Right*; and Gladys Lindberg, founder of the Lindberg Nutrition Service and coauthor with her daughter Judy Lindberg McFarland of *Take Charge of Your Health*.

Nathan Pritikin

Nathan Pritikin, engineer by profession, educated himself thoroughly in nutrition and degenerative disease. He dedicated his life to helping persons find new health and longer life through his diet and exercise program, particularly persons with heart disease. He established the Longevity Center in Santa Barbara, California, and the Longevity Research Institute. Thousands of people have benefited from the Pritikin program. Senator George McGovern, at Pritikin's funeral, eulogized, "Nathan Pritikin was a man of great dedication, unusual humility, a bold pioneer, perhaps the greatest lifesaver that lived in the twentieth century."[1] Yet later research has revealed nutritional elements that were lacking in the Pritikin diet—namely the vital importance of quality fats in the diet to provide the essential fatty acids that help to protect the body against both heart disease and cancers. These missing elements are outlined in *Beyond Pritikin*. Pritikin did not understand the vital role of essential fatty acids in maintaining health. Thus he resorted to drug treatment for his leukemia. But he was so disillusioned that he committed suicide.

Adele Davis

Adele Davis's work in nutrition was ahead of most of the current health literature. For many years her books were the primary nutrition instruction for millions of people. Yet Ms. Davis died of bone cancer. She attributed the disease partly to her habit of smoking which she stopped two years before her death. Faced with sickness and death, Ms. Davis gave her life to Jesus Christ.

Gladys Lindberg

Gladys Lindberg spent over 40 years of her life sharing the benefits of good nutrition to better the lives of millions of people. Adele Davis was one of her lifelong friends. Mrs. Lindberg writes in *Take Charge of Your Health*: "During her illness, I visited her frequently, and she, knowing my relationship with God, asked many penetrating questions. At last, she asked to be taken to a special religious service, and that day I saw this great lady surrender her life to Jesus Christ."[2]

For Nathan Pritikin, health was an end in itself. It was his life pursuit. When he learned that he no longer possessed it, he had nothing left for which to live. For Adele Davis, suffering from a degenerative disease was used by God to get her attention. She responded and recognized that physical health is not all there is to life. Gladys Lindberg ministered to more than Ms. Davis's physical need. Her loving friendship and faith in the Lord Jesus Christ opened the door for Ms. Davis. "Now this is eternal life: that they may know you, the only true God, and Jesus Christ, whom you have sent" (John 17:3).

God has given His children a mission in the world to reconcile people to the one true God through Jesus Christ. While Nathan Pritikin and Adele Davis ministered the benefits of God's natural law to others in the healthy years of their lives, neither was able to bring the life of God in Christ to people. The greatest glory of Ms. Davis's life was her recognition of Jesus Christ as her Lord and Savior. Yet, Gladys Lindberg's healthy life has been used of God not only to teach people how to use His whole food resources for better health, but also to introduce them to the Life-giver!

Why then should we concern ourselves with health? We are concerned so we can better minister the life that is in Christ to a hurting and hungry world. "For we are God's workmanship, created in Christ Jesus to do good works, which God prepared in advance for us to do" (Ephesians 2:10). Our God-given ministries and good works are many and varied. We need all the physical, mental, and emotional strength that food and other good habits of living can supply to carry out these tasks.

41

The Perfect Vegetarian Diet in the New Age

———— ♥ ————

Have nothing to do with godless myths and old wives' tales; rather, train yourself to be godly. For physical training is of some value, but godliness has value for all things, holding promise for both the present life and the life to come.

1 Timothy 4:7,8

———— ♥ ————

There is a growing army of sincere Christians who are enthusiastic advocates of vegetarianism, and there are Christians who avoid it altogether because of its associations with Eastern cultic religious philosophy. There is a difference between a vegetarian diet practiced for nutritional reasons and cultic "vegetarianism." If we are vegetarian enthusiasts, we need to be fully aware of its cultic implications. And if we are skeptics, we must take care not to shun the nutritional value of a potentially nutritious diet.

From the nutritional standpoint the vegetarian diet is much to be preferred over the American Diet. We have already defined vegetarian diets (p. 52). We have introduced both problems of meat-eating and of dairy products, and discussed the merits of the complex carbohydrates as our best foods in other chapters.

Cultic vegetarianism, on the other hand, is a religious practice that denies the Lordship of Jesus Christ, and is antibiblical. For example the "ultimate perfection of a vegetarian diet" is "eating only food offered to Kṛṣṇa."[1] The cultic vegetarian who aims for this perfection will offer his food as a sacrifice to Kṛṣṇa before he eats it. Such food offered to Kṛṣṇa is called "*prasadam,* a Sanskrit word meaning 'mercy of the Lord.'"[2] We must not think that this "Lord" is our Lord Jesus! It is not! Christians can easily be misled by the concepts of cultic vegetarianism because not only is "the Lord" spoken of freely, but arguments from the Bible to prove vegetarianism are used. It is easy for us to be fooled if we are not discerning of the spirits. These arguments from Scripture are incomplete. For example, religious vegetarians will use them to "prove" that our Lord was a vegetarian, but they overlook such key incidents as Jesus feeding the 5000 men with five loaves of barley bread and two fish (John 6:1-15), Jesus providing a large catch of fish for the disciples on two different occasions (Luke 5:4-6 and John 21:5,6), Jesus serving them fish for breakfast Himself (John 21:13), and eating fish Himself (Luke 24:40-43). In addition, the fact that Jesus fulfilled all the Old Testament law during His earthly life means that He inevitably partook of the lamb served yearly at the Jewish Passover feast.

Cultic vegetarians also twist the meaning of Genesis 9:4, "But you must not eat meat that has its lifeblood still in it," to mean that God commanded man not to eat meat at all. This is a direct contradiction of Genesis 9:3: "Everything that lives and moves will be food for you. Just as I gave you the green plants, I now give you everything." In addition, cultic vegetarians overlook the fact that God instituted the killing of animals as sacrifices for sin before the coming of Christ and that portions of the sacrificial meat and grain offerings were the dietary mainstay of the Levites who served God in performing the sacrifices (Leviticus 7:35,36). Certainly there were restrictions such as not eating the fat and the blood (Leviticus 3:17) and not eating several "unclean" animals forbidden for food (Leviticus 11), but even a weak case for nonmeat eating cannot be made from the Word of God!

Food that is acceptable to the cultic vegetarian must be sacrificed to Krsna: "the material substance of food . . . becomes completely spiritualized."[3] Such spiritualized food, or *prasadam*, is supposedly helpful in achieving the goal of reawakening the soul's original relationship with God.[4] "The very simplest form of offering is to simply pray, 'My dear Lord Krsna, please accept this food.'"[5] We can see that cultic vegetarianism is clearly a denial of Jesus' proclamation, "No one comes to the Father except through me" (John 14:6). The cultic vegetarian preaches a false Christ.

The theology of cultic vegetarianism does not correspond with scientific observation in the field of nutrition, either. For example, according to cultic vegetarian theology, food is not classified according to carbohydrate, protein, fat, or its vitamin and mineral content—things that can be explained and observed by the rational mind. It is classified according to "goodness, passion, and ignorance."[6] "Milk products, sugar, vegetables, fruits, nuts, and grains are foods in the mode of goodness and may be offered to Krsna."[7] Meat, fish, eggs, garlic, and onions are not acceptable to Krsna.[8] Nor is food cooked "by people who are not devotees of Krsna. According to the subtle laws of nature, the cook acts upon the food not only physically, but mentally as well. Food thus becomes an agency for subtle influences on our consciousness."[9]

We may think that this information is irrelevant to our interest in food, but we need to understand that while vegetarianism may have nutritional merit, the basis of its origin is not the Judeo-Christian tradition but Eastern Hinduistic religion that denies the gospel of Christ.* Cultic vegetarianism fits 1 Timothy 4:1-3 exactly: "The Spirit clearly says that in later times some will abandon the faith and follow deceiving spirits and things taught by demons. Such teachings come through hypocritical liars, whose consciences have been seared as with a hot iron. They forbid people to marry and order them to abstain from certain foods, which God created to be received with thanksgiving by those who believe and who know the truth."

---

* An eye-opening mini-education on the relationship between Hinduism, New Age concepts, and vegetarianism can be obtained by reading former Hindu Rabi Maharaj's life story, *Death of a Guru* (see Recommended Reading, p. 381). An invaluable book!

42

The Great New Age Health Deception

———— ♥ ————

The health food boom of the 60's that served up bean sprouts and tofu salads along with exercise has been infused with a sacred side.

Carol McGraw
Los Angeles Times

———— ♥ ————

*I*n the last chapter we discussed cultic vegetarianism, just one aspect of the New Age philosophy. New Age philosophy is based on the concept that God and man are one. Man has limitless potential that can be realized through tapping into all manner of supernatural sources. All is seen as good and useful to developing human potential. The purpose of developing human potential is self-realization.

What does this have to do with healthy eating? Much, in every way! Adopting a healthy diet can be approached in two different ways. One way is biblical. The other way is diabolical. This may seem like a strong term to use, but it is important to understand the difference.

The biblical foundation for the *Eating Better Lifestyle* is based on two truths: 1) The God of the Bible—Yahweh, Jehovah—the God of Abraham, Isaac, and Jacob is Creator and Sustainer of the Universe; and 2) the same God is the Redeemer through His Son, Jesus Christ. It is from Him, and Him alone that we draw our resources for life, both natural and supernatural. Our purpose is not to find self-realization but to obey Jesus Christ.

What has happened in the New Age Movement is this: People have begun looking for answers to ultimate health. One thing leads to another. Diet alone is not sufficient. More is needed. There is a whole world of supernatural benefits, as well, to tap into. For example, the theme of the Whole Life Expo held in Pasadena, California, from February 6–8, 1987, was "Explore New Frontiers of Health and Self." The expo offered numerous seminars and workshops on how to utilize these supernatural avenues for health, along with the usual food and diet emphasis.

"They are becoming involved in a world of evil and ultimately in the whole realm of Satan's jurisdiction,"[1] says F. LaGard Smith, author of *Out on a Broken Limb*. An "almost common experience in American society"[2] today is delving into such realms as witchcraft, astrology, clairvoyance, mediumship, metaphysical counseling, trance channeling, astro-travel, crystals, and reincarnation. According to Andrew Greely, "four in ten Americans say they have had contact with the dead and 60% have experienced extrasensory perception."[3] The Christian rejects all supernatural avenues to health that God has forbidden in His Word. We have but one supernatural avenue: the Holy Spirit who lives in us.

Many diets assume a nonbiblical philosophy. We must be careful to distinguish between nutritional value and religious trappings. For example, one of the coauthors of a well-researched and influential cookbook wrote:

A mantram, very simply, is a name of the Lord, hallowed by the thousands of people who have repeated it. People have used some form of mantram in almost all the great religious traditions. "Jesus, Jesus" is a mantram; "Rama, Rama" is Gandhi's mantram. It seems paradoxical, but repeating the mantram has a way of keeping you planted firmly in the right here and right now, concentrated and calm. Not only that, but it helps you to remember all the while that you aren't just slapping together a meal; you're preparing food for the Lord in those you love.[4]

There is a proliferation of such antibiblical philosophy propagated throughout health-food stores, cooking classes, television cooking shows, university extension classes, health magazines, health and nutrition books, cookbooks, and by health practitioners. We can easily be deceived because these resources 1) communicate much sound nutritional information; 2) use Christian terminology when speaking of "the Lord"; 3) work for the same apparent goals as Christianity such as peace and love; and 4) use the ploy that "It works." Christians have been especially drawn in by this latter philosophy, "It works." On the surface it appears innocent enough. But Christians must ask, "Is it based on what is biblically true?" It is easy to embark on a healthier lifestyle without understanding the basis for it. This is dangerous. There is more at stake than physical health. There is no way to have true or eternal peace and love, for example, except through faith in Jesus Christ. Every good work of our lives must be built upon that foundation—including the physical and practical matters such as diet.

43

Give Thanks

———— ♥ ————

*For everything God created is good, and nothing is to
be rejected if it is received with thanksgiving, because it
is consecrated by the word of God and prayer.*

1 Timothy 4:4,5

———— ♥ ————

"Bless this food to the nourishment of our bodies."
Do we pray this prayer as a traditional hangover
from Grandpa's generation or do we really mean it? Do we
think that our prayer will somehow transform the nutritional value of the food? The word *consecrated* in the
dictionary is defined as "set apart or dedicated to the service of the deity." When we give thanks for our food to
God, our Creator and Redeemer, we acknowledge that He
has created it and given it to us as a gift.

If we give thanks to God because He created the food
for our nourishment, how important is it that it retain its
nutrient value? If we give thanks to Him for giving it to us
as a gift, is it right to turn the gift into something it wasn't
meant to be? Let's be honest. We may be able to continue to

give thanks to God for devitalized food in ignorance. But once we know what true nutritional food value is, can we honestly give thanks for inferior food when we know we could do better?

Let's be clear about one thing: Giving thanks for our food does not change its nutritional value, nor does it change the way our bodies will process it. Giving thanks from the heart to God is a health-giving action in itself, but it does not affect the physical nature of the food.

Everything God created is good. Our perversion of many of His good things is not cause for thanksgiving, but for repentance and change. Let us consecrate to His service food that reflects His creative purpose for it—our health and well-being for His honor and glory.

44

Dealing with Opposition

———— ♥ ————

*Let us not become weary in doing good, for at the
proper time we will reap a harvest if we do not give up.*

Galatians 6:9

———— ♥ ————

"*A*re we going to have that weird stuff again, Mom?"
"Here comes the health nut . . . I wonder what she
brought this time!" "Is she trying to kill us?" "Gee, can't we
go to McDonald's for dinner?"

You are convinced that the *Eating Better Lifestyle* is important for your family. You readily began the challenge
with plenty of resources. You thought you were following
all the "dos" of a winsome approach. Bam! The opposition
comes. Are you ready for it? No matter how well and how
carefully you pursue your plan, you will receive some negative responses. Your children may complain, your husband
may be indifferent, friends may tease you, relatives may be
offended, others may give you the cold shoulder. You know
that what you are doing is right. You have done your research and made your commitment to God.

222

Why the opposition?

We travel a narrow road. The world food system consists of two approaches, both of them unbalanced—the hedonistic and the restrictive. The hedonistic approach to food is the American Diet sold to the public by big food corporations who don't care about your health unless it means more profit. Most of the profit is made by appealing to the lusts of the flesh, however. The restrictive approach challenges us with: "Don't use any salt. Don't use eggs. Don't use butter. Don't use honey. Don't eat fish. Don't use dairy products. Don't, don't, don't!" How can you weather the storms of criticism?

First, be fully convinced that developing the *Eating Better Lifestyle* is God's purpose for you based on the foundation of the Scriptures and on sound nutritional information. Be adaptable to changes as new nutritional information is brought to light and as you further understand the Scriptures. Second, find the support of another person. Third, bring each obstacle to God in prayer as it comes. Request His guidance for a workable solution and for His power to transform attitudes. Trust God to assist your efforts. Be on the alert for possible problems you may be causing yourself through a wrong approach or attitude. Sometimes God says "wait." If that happens, wait and watch. Pray for the barriers to be broken and watch for the appropriate opportunities to begin anew. Do not give up because you meet opposition. It is the normal condition of a godly life.

45

Prayer and Fasting

———— ♥ ————

Is not this the kind of fasting I have chosen: to loose the chains of injustice and untie the cords of the yoke, to set the oppressed free and break every yoke?

Isaiah 58:6

———— ♥ ————

The *Eating Better Lifestyle* is not complete without the discipline of prayer and fasting.

Fasting is "the ultimate" in convenience and economy! What a respite from the kitchen! Even most children can fast safely up to 24 hours, especially if fresh fruit juices are substituted for water. If the rest of the family must eat, or is unwilling to fast, you—chief cook and bottle washer—can let them eat a freezer casserole while you fast. Even if you are the only one fasting one day a week, you will realize a savings of $150 to $200 on the yearly food budget. You might make a plan to contribute the money saved to feed the hungry.

Many of us experience unpleasant side effects of fasting

(even for a day) that will obstruct our work. This usually happens because our bodies are not healthy enough to sustain a fast with only water. The body is in need of cleansing from toxins. If this is your experience, fast with fresh fruit juice (see p. 175).

Sue benefits periodically from an excellent juice fast. She puts ³/₈ cup pure maple syrup and ³/₈ cup lemon juice in a quart jar and fills it up with distilled water, then stirs in a little over ¹/₈ teaspoon cayenne pepper. She sets a timer to remind herself to drink the juice, spacing her drinks throughout the day. The lemon juice cleanses the body of toxins. The maple syrup provides valuable energy and the nutrients she needs to sustain health and energy. The cayenne pepper is a blood cleanser and also prevents the drink from having a "sickening" sweet taste. For a full cleansing effect, a ten-day fast on this juice is recommended. Drink about six-and-a-half 10-oz. glasses (two quarts) of this a day. You can drink up to 12 glasses a day, but not less than 6. Forget about the calories—they are not important. A time of fasting is a good time to choose a special verse or passage of Scripture to memorize (see Jeremiah 15:16; Psalm 119:103).

Most persons can safely fast once a week for 24 to 36 hours. Fasting gives the body an extended rest from digestion, helps to cleanse the body of toxic wastes, and serves to clear the cobwebs from the mind. A period of fasting can break a craving for a particular food, especially if the fast is of three days' duration or longer. A periodic fast of three days, three or four times a year, is safe for most people.

Fasting provides a special opportunity for communion with God. It is a time to do spiritual battle to break through seemingly impossible barriers in your own or someone else's life.

To learn how to fast and how to prepare for problems that may arise during a fast, read at least one of the following (see Recommended Reading, pp. 379-80):

God's Chosen Fast by Arthur Wallis

Greater Health God's Way by Stormie Omartian

In regard to fasting for weight control, review p. 164.

46

Good Food Is Good for Love

---------- ♥ ----------

Better a meal of vegetables where there is love than a fattened calf with hatred.

Proverbs 15:17

---------- ♥ ----------

*M*ealtimes are the best times for family fellowship and communication. Children need family relationships expressed in the context of eating together. A survey was taken to discover what high school valedictorians had in common. One activity was found: Each ate one meal a day together with the family. Sue's family followed this mealtime practice. Two of her children graduated from high school with a 4.0 grade point average. The third graduated as valedictorian. One graduated summa cum laude and another magna cum laude from college. Meals shared say "I love you" when Jesus Christ is the center of our relationships. They bind families together.

It is not easy for a family to enjoy quality meals to-gether. The pervasive influences oppose it. The average American child views 8,500 to 13,000 food commercials on television per year—23 to 36 per day![1] The restaurant in-dustry spent $930 million on advertising in 1984. Advertis-ing has made deep inroads on the Christian family. We are so busy working to earn a living and doing "work for the Lord" in the name of Christian ministry, we have yielded the decisions about food value to the profit makers of our society. We have been sold a new value system based on taste, eye appeal, convenience, and nutritional half-truths. Approximately 42% of meals are now eaten away from home. The number of families who eat together even one meal a day is diminishing at an alarming rate.

What we have done in our churches with the Lord's Supper (communion) is illustrative of our disregard for the central place that food can have in living the gospel of Jesus Christ. We now pass the wafer and the grape juice while our pastors illuminate their meaning from the Word of God. Yet our Lord instituted the Lord's Supper in the context of the Jewish Passover meal. The first-century Christians cel-ebrated it in the context of mealtimes. The essence of Jesus' death was not just expressed in a sermon, but experienced in the fellowship, communion, and intimacy of eating to-gether. The "visible" food was an expression of the "invis-ible" nature of God. Romans 1:20 and Psalm 19:1-4 clearly express that God reveals His glory in physical realities. How then can we enhance the meaning of the gospel of Christ both in our own lives and to the world through our use of food? There are many wonderful ways!

Sharing the Gospel of Jesus Christ Through Food

Sharing healthful food is basic to a full expression of God's love. The unhealthy American Diet that leads to sick-ness and premature death is not in harmony with the life-giving gospel of Jesus Christ. "If Jesus truly nourishes us and the Lord's Supper is to remind us of that, we should eat food that truly nourishes."[2] The wife of Proverbs 31 was a businesswoman. She was a busy woman. Yet she did not neglect the affairs of her household. She brought her husband "good, not harm, all the days of her life" (Proverbs 31:12). She brought her food from afar and provided food for her family (31:14,15). To do so today requires a careful selection of health-producing food for our spouses and our children, and also for every person with whom we share food. To offer any other kind of food is an incomplete expression of love.

"There is nothing that says lovin' like something from the oven," is one food commercial that speaks truth. Food can express love in a way that a thousand words cannot. Our Lord said, "Anyone who gives you a cup of water in my name because you belong to Christ will certainly not lose his reward" (Mark 9:41). He placed high value on physical provisions offered in His name. When food is shared in the name of Jesus Christ, it is not a mere excuse for evangelism. It is the gospel in action. There are many occasions for sharing food.

Every important celebration includes food: birthdays, weddings, funerals. Compassion and kindness can be extended with food to the new neighbor, to a neighbor moving elsewhere, to a family with illness or the arrival of a new baby, to a family experiencing a death, to a friend or neighbor who is out of a job, or to the poor in the community. Churches enjoy having coffees, potlucks, fellowship meals, Sunday school refreshments, women's luncheons, men's prayer breakfasts, and picnics. Some fellowships participate in organized food ministries to the poor, to the sick, and to shut-ins.

These occasions do not require high-fat, low-fiber, devitalized food. Proverbs 15:17 explains why we do not need it: "Better a meal of vegetables where there is love . . ." This means that healthy eating is not merely a private affair. It is not something to set aside on the way to the church potluck. We do not need to reform the church by edict or by law about food. But we can each begin to introduce whole foods to believers through informal food-sharing opportunities. Moving the *Eating Better Lifestyle* out of our homes into public ministry in our churches and among friends and neighbors will not be easy. Many of us will be alone in our endeavors and often misunderstood, even teased or ridiculed—yes, even by fellow Christians! Yet such a commitment to the life-giving value of food is essential to the life-giving ministries of the church. We need a "vision." Our growing awareness and pioneer efforts in sharing whole foods with others in all of these various situations can be forerunners pointing to the ministry of the church worldwide to people who are hungry, both physically and spiritually, which we will discuss in the next chapter.

If you are a leader in your church fellowship—pastor, elder, deacon, deaconess, women's ministries leader, hospitality chairperson, head of a food outreach ministry, youth director who plans youth outings and parties, a camp food manager—ask God to give you a "vision" for bringing the life-giving nutritional value of food to the ministry for which you are responsible. Pastors, elders, and husbands who are not involved with food preparation need to understand the role of food in the gospel of Jesus Christ and begin to support those who are becoming nutritionally aware.

The mark of the church is the love of Jesus Christ expressed in ministries to hurting people. Peggy is a person "hurting" from a compulsive chocolate addiction. The church, on the one hand, offers ministries to persons like Peggy for coping with and conquering compulsive behavior. On the other hand, when Peggy finds chocolate brownies served at a church gathering she says, "It is like going to an Alcoholics Anonymous meeting and finding a bar there." We all love chocolate brownies, but we have disregarded the health needs of many brothers and sisters.

Food Sharing Opportunities

Jewish Feast Celebrations: Many Christians are reviving the celebration of Jewish feasts with a Christian interpretation—the Passover seder in the spring, the Feast of Tabernacles in the fall, and others. The Feast of Tabernacles can be celebrated in lieu of our American Thanksgiving (for information write *Eating Better with Sue* (p. 383). *Celebrate the Feasts* by Martha Zimmerman is an excellent resource. *Eating Better Lifestyle* recipes are easily adaptable to these celebrations.

Lord's Supper Celebration: Communion can be shared in the context of a meal with fellow church members in homes or in the church fellowship hall periodically. Whole-wheat matzos could be served in place of communion bread or wafers made with white flour. See *Loaves & Fishes* (Recommended Reading, p. 380) for an agape menu.

Potluck for the Poor: Share an inexpensive soup and muffin meal as a church fellowship periodically and take an offering for the poor or for a Chrisitan organization that ministers to the needy (such as World Vision or World Relief Commission).

Anniversary or Wedding: Serve a whole-wheat wedding cake with cream cheese frosting. The decoration can be made with regular decorator icing. One of Sue's friends enjoyed a three-tiered wedding cake for 250 persons prepared from the Applesauce Cake in *Eating Better Desserts* (see p. 384 for information). Serve a trail mix, punch with real fruit juice, and vegetable relish tray with dip. The groom's cake can be whole-wheat banana bread or fruitcake.

Birthday or Children's Parties: Serve whole-wheat cake or cupcakes, real fruit juice punch, whole-grain cookies, and frozen yogurt or honey vanilla ice cream.

New Neighbor: Take a loaf of homemade whole-wheat bread or muffins in a colorful basket.

Death in a Family: Skip desserts and take something basic so that those who are grieving do not need to cook, such as hearty soup, muffins, a main dish salad, a casserole dish. Sue did not have to cook any meals for a full week following the death of her son, Stephen. Love shared in this way is a great blessing.

Unemployment: Share a "love basket" of something you prepare yourself or produce from the garden—a loaf of fresh bread, muffins, a pound of butter, a jar of honey, a batch of granola. Many do not appreciate handouts, so make it something fun and special rather than a basic bag of groceries until you discern the recipients' feelings. Then, if basic groceries are appreciated, make them better-quality items such as fertile eggs, water-pack tuna, Hollywood mayonnaise, peanut butter without hydrogenated fat and sugar, etc.

Home Schooling: The home school setting is a wonderful opportunity to learn about preparing and serving whole foods with children. Parents can learn at the same time (see pp. 77-78).

Restaurant Meal: Take a small loaf of homebaked whole-wheat bread to give to the waitress with a note of appreciation attached for her services.

Love Basket: All Christian marriages need rekindling with romantic moments. Fill a love basket for an overnight or a day's outing with favorite whole foods.

Church Coffees, Potlucks, Classes, etc.: Offer whole-food alternatives. For example, serve herb teas alongside the coffee, real fruit juice in place of punch, fresh fruits or whole-grain home-baked goods alongside commercial doughnuts and cookies.

Meals from Bible Times: As an evangelistic outreach to friends and neighbors, host a series of meals from Bible times, sharing informally the historical context of each one. Invite the guests to participate in a home Bible study. Use *Loaves & Fishes* for menus and historical resources (see Recommended Reading, p. 380).

If you take a tasty dish to a potluck such as a dozen *Minute Blender Bran Muffins,* you'll influence 12 people with how tasty whole foods can really be. You will even get requests for recipes!

47

Christian Ministry in a Hungry World

---- ♥ ----

For he satisfies the thirsty and fills the hungry with good things.

Psalm 107:9

---- ♥ ----

The train lurched to a stop in the Mexican village. Young girls rushed forward and eagerly held bags of succulent mangoes up to our window. Imposing itself on the landscape behind them loomed a Coca-Cola truck—the only vehicle in sight parked on the single muddy village street. That one scene captured the reality of what is happening worldwide. People everywhere are being inundated by refined, devitalized food.

Wherever refined foods such as soda pop, white flour and white sugar products, polished white rice, and canned foods have traveled, the health of people has deteriorated. Cavities and crooked teeth, diabetes, heart disease, cancer, and obesity are the legacies of refined food. Research projects conducted worldwide bear out the truth of this fact consistently. Says D.B. Jelliffe in *Nutritional Reviews*, September 1972, "The food industry in developing countries has been a disaster . . . a minus influence."[1]

Why is this happening? It is happening because powerful food industries are expanding their marketing of refined food products throughout the world. People in other countries are just as interested in convenience foods as are Americans. Food from the West is also viewed as a status symbol. In Africa, for example, many will shun the local whole grains in favor of white rice.

The food industry not only influences the nutritional quality of food throughout the world, but it also influences the economics and politics of supply. There is ample food to feed the world. Natural disasters and lack of land to grow food may appear to be the reasons for hunger, but they are not. The Institute of Food and Development Policy cites economics and politics as the root causes of hunger.

Why should Christians be concerned? The same influences that have created the devitalized condition of our food supply in America are traveling across the world. Many Christians travel throughout the world to take the gospel of Jesus Christ to other people. Most missionaries take the influences of the refined American Diet with them. In contrast, missionaries Charles and Edna Lewis have chosen to take full advantage of the local whole foods where they live. As a result, Charles can do the work of four local Christian men because he eats a nutritious diet. In addition, the Lewises have opportunity to share with their friends the best use of the locally available whole foods. It is food for thought.

A real eye-opener on how our Western diet has affected the rest of the world is *Nutrition and Physical Degeneration* by Weston A. Price, D.D.S. (see Recommended Reading, p. 381). In the 1930s and 1940s, Dr. Price visited over 130 people groups throughout the world in every type of geographical location. He studied these peoples in terms of dental health before and after the influence of Western diet practices. What he learned is astounding—and tragic. Accompanying the text are over 200 "before and after" photos. Sue considers this book "must" reading for missionaries.

48

Food for Thought

———— ♥ ————

When your words came, I ate them: they were my joy and my heart's delight, for I bear your name, O LORD God Almighty.

Jeremiah 15:16

———— ♥ ————

Take 15 minutes a week around the family dinner table to read and discuss portions of Scripture about food. The list below is not exhaustive, but provides a wealth of information. You might enjoy preparing some of the meals (using ingredients of higher nutritional quality, where needed) from *Loaves & Fishes: Foods from Bible Times* by Malvina Kinard and Janet Crisler (see Recommended Reading, p. 380). These meals will bring some of the food customs you read about to life.

Food in the Bible

God, the Provider
Genesis 1:29
Genesis 27:28
Exodus 16
Deuteronomy 8:10-18
Psalm 85:11,12
Psalm 104:14,27,28

Vegetarianism Issue
(as an authoritative standard)
Genesis 4:2-5
Genesis 9:3
Exodus 12:1-11
Deuteronomy 12:20-25
1 Kings 17:6
Luke 22:7,8
Luke 24:41-43
John 6:11
John 21:5-13
Romans 14:6-8
1 Timothy 4:1-5

Vegetarian Diet
(as a personal choice)
Daniel 1:8-16
Proverbs 15:17
Romans 14:3,4
1 Corinthians 6:12

Meat
Genesis 9:3,4
Genesis 18:1-8
Leviticus 7:22,23,26
Leviticus 7:28-36
Leviticus 11
Deuteronomy 32:14
Acts 15:22-29

Judging Eating Preferences
Romans 14

Rich Food; Gluttony
Proverbs 17:1
Proverbs 23:1-3
Proverbs 23:20,21
Proverbs 28:7
Titus 1:11,12

Grains
Genesis 41:56–42:2
Deuteronomy 8:8
Deuteronomy 32:14
Ruth 2
Isaiah 28:23-29

Food Lists
Genesis 43:11
Deuteronomy 8:7-9
Deuteronomy 32:13,14
1 Samuel 25:18
2 Samuel 17:28,29

Honey
Numbers 14:7,8
Deuteronomy 32:13
Proverbs 24:13
Proverbs 25:16,27
1 Samuel 14:24-29
Isaiah 7:14,15
Isaiah 7:22
Mark 1:6

Eggs
Job 6:6
Luke 11:11,12

Salt
Job 6:6
Matthew 5:13
Colossians 4:6

Oil
Deuteronomy 8:8
Deuteronomy 32:13
1 Kings 17:7-16
Proverbs 21:17,20

Butter, Curds, Cream
Genesis 18:8
Deuteronomy 32:14
Judges 5:25
Proverbs 30:33
Isaiah 7:14,15
Isaiah 7:21,22

Milk
Genesis 18:1-8
Numbers 14:7,8
Deuteronomy 32:14
Judges 4:19
Proverbs 27:27
Isaiah 55:1
Ezekiel 25:4
Joel 3:18
1 Corinthians 9:7

Bread of Affliction
(not a recipe for pleasure)
Ezekiel 4:9-13

Care of the Body
Romans 12:1,2
1 Corinthians 6:12,13
1 Corinthians 6:19,20

*Home Management and
Teaching Children*
Genesis 1:28
Psalm 8:3-8
Psalm 115:16
Psalm 127:1
Proverbs 14:1
Proverbs 14:27
Proverbs 31:10-12
Proverbs 31:14,15
Proverbs 31:26,27
Hosea 4:6
Titus 2:4,5
2 Peter 1:5-7

Food Cost
Isaiah 55:2

An Unworthy Meal
Genesis 27:7-34
Hebrews 12:16

An Energizing Meal
1 Kings 19:5-8

An Eternal Meal
John 6:1-14

PART 6

Action

49

Planning Is a Privilege

———— ♥ ————

*Command those who are rich in this present world not
to be arrogant nor to put their hope in wealth, which is
so uncertain, but to put their hope in God, who richly
provides us with everything for our enjoyment.*

1 Timothy 6:17

———— ♥ ————

The Israelites in the wilderness complained bitterly to
Moses: "If only we had died by the LORD's hand in
Egypt! There we sat around pots of meat and ate all the food
we wanted, but you have brought us out into this desert to
starve this entire assembly to death" (Exodus 16:3). How
quickly they forgot about their slavery in Egypt and the
power of God to deliver them. You may be wondering, too,
as you develop the *Eating Better Lifestyle*, "Is it worth it all?"

The Israelites were consigned to 40 years of eating
manna for their lack of faith in God's ability to provide for
them. Each day they were to collect what manna they
needed—no gardening, no harvesting, no storing of food,

no grocery shopping, no menu planning, no food preparation, no recipes to follow. Just the same thing to eat meal after meal—"manna waffles, manna burgers . . . ba-manna bread . . ."![1] If we lived in a developing country, our food variety could be limited and scarce. Which would we rather have—starvation rations, only one or two foods to eat, or an abundance that requires planning and discipline? Let us bless our God—not with complaints, but with thankful hearts for the abundance we must manage!

50

Meal Planning and Shopping

———— ♥ ————

Make plans by seeking advice. . . .
Proverbs 20:18

———— ♥ ————

"*H*elp! I've never been so bogged down and frustrated with meals, time, energy, and finances in my life. Everything has run away with me. I'm a wife, a mother of four children, a nurse attending a community college, and active in our local church. But meals become a real headache. At 5:00 P.M. I fall apart. HELP! HELP!"

We often receive a letter like this from busy moms. Meal planning can save headaches, stress, and even finances in homes. Emilie knows from the experience of feeding five children under five years of age, one husband, and many drop-in friends, family, and hungry people. Sue knows from feeding family, live-in students, and hundreds of campers. Mealtime can and will be a joy when, and only when, we plan ahead! It takes little time to save much time. *Have a plan, work the plan, and the plan will work for you.*

How to Plan Meals

Keep your meal plan simple by focusing only on the dinner menus for one week. First make a simple chart: Fold an 8½" x 11" sheet of paper in half lengthwise. Fold it in half crosswise and in half again crosswise. You now have eight squares. Write a day of the week in seven of the squares.* Select a main dish for each square. Start with our Unlimited Meal Plan or No-Meat or No-Dairy No-Egg meal plans (pp. 309-11). Choose one to three new recipes. You can choose more, but don't overdo it. Space these new recipes between your regular familiar meals. After you have written in the main dishes you can add choices of vegetables, salads, and breads.

When you have finished the meal chart, decide on a few ingredient changes you can start making in your own favorite dishes. Choose from the list of Super Starter Steps (chapter 52). Note these on the chart. For example, if you plan to use ground turkey in the spaghetti on Thursday evening, write "with ground turkey" in the Thursday square. If you are going to put darker leafy lettuce in the tossed salad on Monday evening, write "with dark leafy lettuce" under tossed salad in the square. If you are going to make any changes for breakfasts, lunches, or snacks, note them briefly in the eighth blank square on your chart. For example, you may note "new breakfast cereal," "raisins and sunflower seeds for snacks," "whole-wheat bread for toast." Now you are ready to prepare the shopping list.

---

* A complete, simple planning system with charts, plus ten four-week meal plans of 30-61 menus each to meet different needs and interests and 200 menus are available in *Eating Better Cookbooks* (see p. 384 for information).

The Shopping List

Arrange your market list in the same order that food items are arranged in the market where you do most of your shopping. This will take you through the aisles of the market quickly. List all the ingredients needed for your main dishes. Many of the ingredients needed for our recipes can be purchased in the supermarket. Check the Shopping Guide (chapter 54) for a complete list of ingredients used in the recipes in this book. Those that require a health-food store are marked with an asterisk (*). Write the health-food store ingredients on a separate list.

Next, list the necessary fruits, vegetables, dairy products, breads, cereals, condiments, etc. needed for the balance of the dinner meals and for breakfasts and lunches. Include snack foods such as in-season fresh fruits, dates, raw and unsalted nuts, carrots, zucchini (to cut into sticks), celery, cucumbers, and turnip rounds.

Now work on your health-food-store list. You may be making your first trip to a health-food store. Check "How to Locate Shopping Resources" (chapter 59) if you need help in locating one. If you want to begin stocking your pantry with items from the health-food store that are not on your week's meal plan, a beginner list is given on pp. 270-71. In addition, you might want to take the Survey Checklist (pp. 272-75) with you.

Generally, health-food stores are further from home. You can save extra trips later by shopping for staples in advance. But stick to the list of items on pp. 270-71 unless you know exactly what you are going to do with other items you might purchase. Don't do like our friend Jamie, who gave away all her familiar pantry items and completely restocked the kitchen with health-food store products she did not know how to use. When they got bugs in them, she decided that she wasn't ready for that kind of cooking. She tried to do too much at once. Keep things simple. It is better to do one new thing well that will become a way of life than to do too many things and give up in frustration.

Include your family in preparing the weekly meal chart and shopping lists. An older child can note items to purchase as you plan menus with your husband and/or children. Children love eating what they have planned and prepared. This is part of helping the family to change. If you train them well, they can take over for you completely on frequent occasions when they get older (a super time-saving bonus!).

The Shopping Trip

Plan to shop the same day each week. Shopping will be more complex while starting the *Eating Better Lifestyle*. Once you have located your best resources, a pattern will develop. You will probably shop at more than one store—supermarket, health-food store, dairy, local produce stand. You may need to make a second shopping trip during the week for fresh produce. Check the ads in your newspaper. Supermarkets restock periodically each week. Shop when produce items are available in fresh abundance. Eat beforehand so that you are not hungry. Keep to your market list and shop quickly. Women spend at least 75 cents a minute after the first half hour in the market, according to one study. Women who adhere to planned whole-food menus and market lists save as much as $16 to $20 weekly. If you are easily influenced by disruptive children or by their pleas for items not on your list, do not take them. Otherwise, use the time to teach them how to select fresh foods and packaged foods by reading labels (chapter 58). For example, if an item lists sugar as one of the first two or three ingredients, it is high in sugar. Find a similar item that has no sugar listed and show your child the difference. Suggest that together you buy fresh fruit such as bananas and raisins or dates for a no-sugar cereal. Gradually, your children will also understand that a few minor changes can turn the meals into better eating.

Further Help with Meal Planning and Marketing

Be consistent about the time you plan each week's meals just as you are consistent with shopping days. As you progress in developing the *Eating Better Lifestyle*, you will include more of our recipes and menus, and better ingredients in all your meals. We have given you several guidelines to menu planning and resources to help you in your shopping in Part 6. Use them.

51

Guidelines for Balanced Meal Plans

———— ♥ ————

*W*e would all like to know how we can plan meals to include all the nutrients that we need. Will we get enough calcium, enough protein, enough vitamin A, enough iron? The Recommended Dietary Allowances are put neatly into a chart to let the American public know how much of each accepted nutrient has been judged necessary by the National Research Council for normal health. Some nutrition books and cookbooks such as this one also include nutrient data—usually the total calories, fat, protein, and carbohydrates. In addition we include with each recipe (see p. 308) the exchange values, percentage of calories of protein, fat, and carbohydrate, milligrams of cholesterol and sodium, grams of dietary fiber, and approximate cost. For menus, the per-serving total calories, percentage of calories of fat, and approximate cost are given. Vitamin and mineral content are not listed for recipes because the actual amounts are altered by too many variables such as the quality of seed, the quality of soil the food is grown in, and food storage and preparation practices. Other meal-planning tools include the *Dietary Fiber in Foods Chart* (pp. 95-97), *Calorie Chart* (pp. 98-100), and *Best Food Sources of Vitamins and Minerals* (p. 138-43). All of these can help to give the idea of what we are looking for in our food. When it comes to actually planning the meals, however, we need simple and workable guidelines, focusing on the kinds and quantities of foods. We need to understand nutrition, but it is the food that we see, touch, smell, taste, and prepare. Here are three basic guidelines to assist your meal planning and shopping:

1. FOOD GUIDE (pp. 252-53)

2. BASIC MENU PATTERNS (pp. 254-55)

3. MEAL PLANS (pp. 309-11) (for dinners only)

   a. Unlimited Meal Plan

   b. No-Meat Meal Plan (Lacto-Ovo-Vegetarian) (adaptable to No-Egg Meal Plan (Lacto-Vegetarian)

   c. No-Dairy, No-Egg Meal Plan

The Food Guide gives the general picture. The Basic Menu Patterns suggest the specific type of foods to use in menus. The Meal Plans present specific main-dish menus arranged according to the *Eating Better Cookbooks'* simple system of dinner meal planning: Select a specific type of main dish for the same day of the week throughout the month (e.g. rice or grain vegetarian dish on Sundays, ground turkey dish on Mondays, dairy/cheese/vegetarian dish on Tuesdays and Saturdays, fish dish on Wednesdays, vegetarian bean dish on Thursdays, vegetarian potato or chicken dish on Fridays—see sample meal plan, p. 309). This system is adaptable to any desired categorical arrangement of main dishes. It is the key to Sue's simplified meal planning.

FOOD GUIDE

Fresh Vegetables—think LOTS! think MORE, MORE!
  Especially dark leafy greens, cabbage, broccoli
  Especially dark yellow
  Some for lunch
  Some for dinner

Fresh Fruits—think TWO TO FOUR PIECES MINIMUM
  At least one citrus for vitamin C
  One for breakfast
  Best for snack or separate meal

Whole Grains, Beans, and Peas—think MODERATE
  In combinations in main dishes or,
  Bean dish with bread, or
  Grain with milk or cheese
  Breads, cereals, muffins

Nuts and Seeds—think SMALL
  In baking, main dishes, garnishing
  Small snack

Dairy Products—think SMALL TO MODERATE
  Especially low-fat, nonfat, cultured

Eggs—think ONCE/TWICE A WEEK—think
    IN BAKING OKAY

Meats and Poultry—think BITS 'N' PIECES
  In casseroles, stir-fry, occasional "hunk"

Fish—think 1 TO 3 TIMES A WEEK MINIMUM
  Especially fatty ones—salmon, mackerel, tuna
  Lean fish, too (see calorie list, p. 100)

Fats—think TINY
  Butter on breads, oils for salads
  Both for baking
  Think quality for those essential fats!

Sweets—think SPECIAL OCCASION AND TREAT
  Think honey and other more wholesome sugars
  Think whole-grain flours

How much to eat WHEN?

Breakfasts—think SUBSTANTIAL

Lunches—think SMALLER TO MODERATE

Dinners—think SMALLER TO MODERATE
        Think EARLY
        Think FAMILY TOGETHER

Snacks—think 1 OR 2
Midmorning and/or midafternoon
Fresh fruit, protein, vegetable munchie-crunchies
Don't "wing them"—plan them!

Photocopy this for your kitchen bulletin board or refrigerator door:

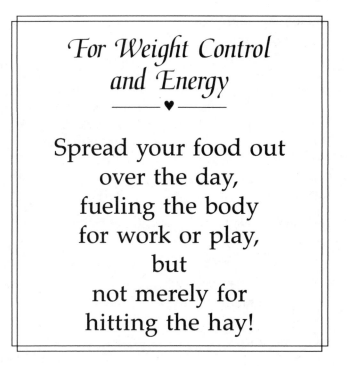

For Weight Control and Energy

♥

Spread your food out
over the day,
fueling the body
for work or play,
but
not merely for
hitting the hay!

BASIC MENU PATTERNS

BREAKFAST PATTERNS:

#1 whole-grain cereal
    low-fat, nonfat milk
      or yogurt
    whole-grain toast
    English muffin, or
      muffin
    fresh fruit piece

#2 egg
    whole-grain toast
    English muffin,
      muffin, or
      coffee cake
    fresh fruit or juice

#3 pancakes/waffles
      or French toast
    fruit topping/
      maple syrup
    yogurt or milk

#4 fresh fruit salad or
      cut fruit wedges
    yogurt or cottage cheese
    crushed nuts, 1-3
      teaspoons

#5 protein shake
    whole-grain toast
      or muffin (optional)

LUNCH PATTERNS:

#1 whole-grain sand-
      wich or pita bread
    high-protein or vegetable
      filling
    dark leafy lettuce
    veggie munchies
    milk or yogurt

#2 soup
    whole-grain muffin
      or crackers
    veggie munchies
    yogurt, cottage
      cheese, or cheddar
      cheese

#3 leafy green salad
    protein bits—egg,
      tuna, chicken, cheese,
      nuts, seeds, beans
    whole-grain muffin,
      bread, or crackers
    milk (optional)

#4 fresh fruit salad or
      cut fruit wedges
    yogurt or cottage
      cheese
    crushed nuts, 1-3
      teaspoons

Lunch Patterns cont.:

#5   protein shake
     whole-grain muffin (optional)

DINNER PATTERNS:

#1   main dish, meatless
     green or veggie salad
     fresh vegetable, cooked
     bread (optional)

#2   main dish with meat
     green or veggie salad
     fresh vegetable, cooked
     bread (optional)

#3   fish, chicken, turkey
     brown rice dish
     green or veggie salad
     fresh vegetable, cooked
     bread (optional)

#4   main dish, cheese
     green salad
     fresh vegetable, cooked
     bread (optional)

#5   soup
     whole-grain muffin
     hot bread/crackers
     veggie munchies or salad
        and/or fresh fruit

#6   fresh fruit salad
     yogurt or cottage cheese
     crushed nuts, 1-3 teaspoons
     whole-grain muffin
        (optional)

#7   protein shake
     whole-grain muffin
        or bread (optional)

#8   egg dish
     green or veggie salad
     fresh vegetable, cooked
     whole-grain muffin, toast,
     or English muffin

#9   large, fresh salad
     high-protein filling
     hot whole-grain bread
        or muffin

ACCOMPANIMENTS: 1½ teaspoons honey, butter, or *Butter Spread* (p. 371), or 1½ teaspoons to 1 tablespoon 100% fruit jam per muffin, roll, or slice of bread; low or nonfat salad dressings or herb vinegar or lemon juice for salads; 1½ teaspoons to 1 tablespoon oil-based dressing per 2 cups or more salad.

52

Super Starter Steps to Improved Meals

———— ♥ ————

$\mathcal{H}$ ere's how to make nutritional improvements in your own favorite meals, many of them by selecting better quality ingredients at the supermarket* and by making simple changes in food preparation.

♥ Begin to replace at least half the iceberg lettuce in tossed salads with darker leafy lettuce such as romaine, green leaf lettuce, or ruby red lettuce. Include at least four other fresh vegetables in tossed salads.

♥ Replace processed cheeses such as American cheese with cheddar, jack, or mozzarella cheese. Try to reduce the amount called for by one-third. Use a

---

* Different brands of better-quality ingredients are sold in different parts of the country. *The Supermarket Handbook* by Nikki and David Goldbeck is an invaluable resource for locating available brands in your area of the country (see Recommended Reading, p. 381).

reduced-fat or reduced or low-sodium cheese, if you can find one that tastes acceptable.

♥ Replace creamed cottage cheese (4% fat) with non-fat or low-fat cottage cheese.

♥ Use ground turkey in place of ground beef in all your favorite burger dishes. Season it before browning (see recipe, p. 320). Use between "90% fat-free" and "99% fat-free" according to your family's taste.

♥ Purchase turkey breakfast sausage in place of pork sausage or bacon for breakfast, or make your own using our *Turkey Sausage* recipe in **Breakfasts** (see p. 384).

♥ In salads and sandwich spreads, replace half the mayonnaise with nonfat or low-fat plain yogurt. Buy mayonnaise that is made without chemical additives or sugar.

♥ Replace sour cream with any of the following combinations, to taste: 1) half sour cream, half nonfat or low-fat yogurt; 2) half nonfat or light sour cream, half nonfat or low-fat yogurt; 3) all nonfat or low-fat yogurt; 4) all nonfat or light sour cream. Use only nonfat or light sour cream in dishes to be frozen.

♥ Use peanut butter made without partially hydrogenated or hydrogenated fat and sugar. Don't get unsalted unless family taste buds enjoy it.

♥ Replace cream cheese with light cream cheese or Neufchatel cheese. Both are lower in fat.

♥ Use long-grain brown rice in place of white rice. If not ready for this, choose Uncle Ben's Converted

Rice in preference to other white rice. More nutrients are retained in processing converted rice. Try mixing half white rice and half brown rice.

♥ Purchase bulgur wheat (also called Ala) to use in any meal in place of rice. Bulgur is parboiled wheat that cooks in a few minutes or may be soaked instead of cooked. Follow package directions. Quinoa (KEEN-Wa) from a health-food store is an interesting alternative. It cooks up in about 20 minutes.

♥ Use half or more whole-wheat flour in baking. Whole-wheat pastry flour, available at health-food stores will produce a lighter texture. Use unbleached white flour for the white flour.

♥ Purchase only whole-grain cold cereals without sugar added such as Shredded Wheat, Grapenuts, NutriGrain cereal, Cheerios. Avoid those that contain partially hydrogenated fat. Health-food stores have many additional choices.

♥ Purchase only whole-grain hot cereals such as Quaker Oats, Wheatena, Zoom, Roman Meal. Health-food stores have many additional choices.

♥ Cut fat in recipes in half, replacing shortening with oil or butter, or with half oil, half butter.

♥ Purchase at least one fresh vegetable from the cabbage family each week to include in the meal plan such as cabbage, broccoli, brussels sprouts, kohlrabi, or cauliflower. There is something in these vegetables that helps to protect against cancer—maybe beta carotene or maybe some other yet unidentified nutrient or combination of them.

♥ Replace distilled vinegar with apple cider vinegar.

♥ Use Kikkoman Milder Soy Sauce to season in place
of soy sauce (unless you are allergic to wheat). One
teaspoon Kikkoman Lite contains 200 mg. sodium
as compared to 314 mg. sodium in regular soy
sauce. Bragg Liquid Aminos, a high-protein soy
product available at health-food stores, is far lower
in sodium than soy sauce and milder in flavor. To
use in a recipe, use more of it, adjusting to taste.

♥ Buy carrots with the tops still attached. Place tops
with ends of spinach, broccoli, parsley, and other
vegetable scraps (saved in a Ziploc bag for a week
or less) in a large pot. Barely cover with water, boil
3 minutes, reduce heat, and simmer 2 hours. Strain
and refrigerate or freeze the broth for use in soups.
This *Vegetable Broth* for soups is demonstrated on
the *"Eating Better with Sue"* video (see p. 383).

♥ Purchase salad dressings with real food ingre-
dients and no sugar or chemical additives, such as
Newman's Own Olive Oil and Vinegar Dressing.
Make our simple dressings, pp. 372-73.

♥ For beef dishes such as stroganoff calling for cubes
or strips, use flank steak. It is the lowest fat beef
cut. Ask butcher to tenderize it for you. Marinate
in one tablespoon Kikkoman Lite Soy Sauce blended
with one tablespoon arrowroot powder (p. 268) or
cornstarch for several hours.

♥ When buying tortilla chips, look for those made
with stoneground cornmeal and vegetable oil that
is not hydrogenated or partially hydrogenated.
Some are also salt-reduced. Some supermarkets
will carry them. Try fat-free baked chips. If not
acceptable to taste, try mixing them half 'n' half
with regular chips. Those made with stoneground
cornmeal, nonhydrogenated oil, reduced or no salt
are much easier to find in health-food stores.

♥ Cut sugar in recipes in half, replacing it with honey. Reduce oven temperature by 25°.

♥ Sauté vegetables in a little water instead of fat.

♥ Cut salt in recipes by one-third and see how they taste. Choose a better quality such as RealSalt, available in some health-food stores, and by mail order (see p. 304).

♥ Use low-fat or nonfat milk instead of whole milk unless it is raw certified milk (see pp. 125-26).

♥ Substitute buttermilk or nonfat yogurt thinned to buttermilk consistency in place of sweet milk in baking. Buttermilk is available at $1/2$% fat, 1% fat, $1^{1}/2$% fat, and 2% fat. Use the lowest percent fat available.

♥ Add more fresh veggies to tuna or egg salad than you usually do—celery, onion, green pepper, cucumber, grated carrot.

♥ Prepare mashed potatoes, potato salad, and fried potatoes without removing skins unless the potato is green just under the skin. This is a toxic substance called solanine. In rare cases a person reacts to glycoalkoids in the skins with headache, diarrhea, or nausea. But most people don't.

♥ Add a few canned kidney and/or garbanzo beans to tossed salad for extra protein, fiber, vitamins, and minerals. Canned beans are high in sodium, but are convenient to use in small amounts. Rinse them well before adding. Rinsing well for 1 minute can remove up to 40% of the sodium. Try "no salt added" or "50% reduced salt" canned beans.

♥ Remove skin from chicken and turkey.

♥ Trim all visible fat from meat and poultry before cooking.

♥ If making a meat, chicken, or turkey broth, refrigerate to let the fat rise to the top. Skim off fat before using.

♥ Buy unsweetened real fruit juices for breakfasts, snacking, and sack lunches (juices without sugar or high fructose corn syrup or sweetener).

♥ Use fresh garlic and fresh onions liberally. Buy a garlic press (see p. 291). One garlic clove replaces ¼ teaspoon garlic powder. An "onion-a-day," raw or cooked, may keep the doctor away better than an apple. Onions are highly effective in facilitating friendly bacteria growth in the intestinal track.

♥ Use garlic powder and onion powder in place of garlic salt and onion salt.

♥ Cut amount of meat called for in a casserole by one-third. Increase the amount of vegetables by one-third.

♥ Purchase at least one bunch of dark leafy greens to include in the meals each week such as kale, collards, spinach, chard, or mustard greens.

♥ Buy everything unsweetened: canned fruits, frozen fruits, canned or boxed juices, frozen juice concentrates, jams, fruit spreads, and jelly. Supermarkets are abundantly supplied with them. Read the ingredients labels carefully. And no aspertame, Equal, or NutraSweet (see p. 150)!

♥ Take a copy of *A Consumer's Dictionary to Food Additives* into the supermarket with you (keep it in the car). See Recommended Reading, p. 379. Don't buy until you've read the ingredients label.

53

How to Improve a Popular American Meal

———— ♥ ————

The menu is:

American Lasagna
(1 serving of 8)

Tossed salad
(2 cups with 1 tablespoon
oil dressing)

Garlic buttered French bread
(2 slices [3 oz.] with
1 tablespoon margarine)

———— ♥ ————

*W*hat can be done to this menu to transform it into an *Eating Better Lifestyle* menu? First, the lasagna— what are the ingredients?

1 lb. lean ground beef	fresh garlic
1 tablespoon oil for frying	tomato paste
salt, pepper, and oregano	canned tomatoes
3 cups creamy cottage cheese	American cheese
8 oz. white flour lasagna noodles	1/2 lb. Swiss cheese

We could omit the ground beef or cut the amount in half and use very lean ground beef—or better, use ground turkey. Omitting the meat altogether would be best, but we'll opt for the ground turkey, pound for pound, and drop the 1 tablespoon fat for frying. Instead of American cheese we might use a little Parmesan cheese, reduce the Swiss by one-third, or substitute mozzarella cheese which has half the fat. The creamy cottage cheese could be replaced by low-fat or nonfat cottage cheese, or skim-milk ricotta. For the white flour lasagna noodles, we'll substitute whole-wheat ones, or we might omit the noodles altogether and make a meatless *Vegetable Lasagna* with zucchini slices, a little onion, some green pepper and fresh mushrooms, a little carrot, a head of steamed and chopped spinach, 1/4 lb. cheese (half mozzarella for less fat), a little Parmesan, and a couple of eggs.

Now for the salad. The average tossed salad consists of iceberg lettuce with a token of red cabbage and tomato wedge topped with more than a sufficient amount of Thousand Island dressing. Why not use half darker leafy lettuce such as romaine, salad bowl, or loose-leaf ruby red and add four or five vegetables not used in the lasagna (except perhaps tomatoes) such as celery, radishes, cucumber, alfalfa sprouts, and jicama? Serve it with olive oil and vinegar dressing, but use half as much; or enjoy a refreshing no-fat salad dressing such as an herb vinegar, a squeeze of lemon juice, or the juice of half an orange (suprisingly tasty on tossed!).

In place of the French bread, serve another vegetable such as cooked broccoli or green beans. Make it a good-sized portion instead of the traditional 1/2 cup. With the lasagna noodles, a bread is not really needed, and with the French bread, the margarine is eliminated, too (in any case, we would use *Butter Spread*). Since there are no noodles in the vegetable lasagna, a bread would be a welcome accompaniment. Why not try something different from the usual, such as delicious baked *Minute Blender Bran Muffins* served with 100 percent fruit jam?

#1—*American Lasagna*
(top of page 264)

#2—*Emilie's Best Lasagna*

2 cups tossed salad	Calories: 33% lower
Sweet Orange Dressing	Fat: 44% lower
1 cup cooked broccoli	Cholesterol: 13% lower
	Sodium: 8% lower
	Dietary Fiber: 267% higher

#3—*Vegetable Lasagna*

2 cups tossed salad	Calories: 16% lower
Sweet Orange Dressing	Fat: 64% lower
2 *Minute Blender Bran Muffins*	Cholesterol: 7% lower
2 tablespoons 100% fruit jam	Sodium: 15% lower
	Dietary Fiber: 467% higher

Our improved menu will be more filling and colorful with more texture interest. With these changes, what have we accomplished nutritionally besides increasing the vitamins and minerals? Let's look at the chart below (for one serving of 8):

Nutrient	#1 American Lasagna	#2 Emilie's Best Lasagna	#3 Vegetable Lasagna
Calories	837	646	698
Protein	35 grams	57 grams	31 grams
Fat	43 grams (47%)	24 grams (31%)	15.5 grams (18%)

Nutrient	#1 American Lasagna	#2 Emilie's Best Lasagna	#3 Vegetable Lasagna
Cholesterol	142 mg.	123 mg.	132 mg.
Sodium	1872	1729	1592
Dietary Fiber	4.5 grams	12 grams	21 grams

We could have done even more! For example, we could have selected lower-sodium tomato products, then seasoned to taste. Check out our lasagna menus, pp. 323, 334—a little different than the menus here, but along the same line. You can similarly transform many typical meals into *Eating Better* meals! Soon you can have meals that will average 40% less fat, cholesterol, and sodium, 220% more dietary fiber, and 25% lower cost than typical American meals!

54

Shopping Guide for Recipes

————— ♥ —————

The following items are used in the recipes in this book. Items that are normally only available at health-food stores are marked with an asterisk (*). Fresh foods (fruits, vegetables, dairy products, tofu, meat, fish, poultry) are not included. All fresh-food ingredients can normally be purchased at the supermarket unless higher-quality organic fresh foods are desired.

Grains, Flours, Pastas, Breads, Cereals:
bran, wheat (unprocessed) (e.g. Miller's Bran)
brown rice, long grain
barley, pearled
*bread, whole-grain sandwich
*cornmeal, stoneground
*corn tortillas, stoneground
*hamburger buns, whole-grain

*lasagna noodles, whole-grain
*millet (p. 355 only)
*noodles, whole-grain
oat bran
oats, rolled
*spaghetti, whole-grain
*whole-wheat pastry flour (preferred) or whole-wheat flour
*whole-wheat tortillas

267

Beans, Dry:
black-eyed peas
lentils
mixed beans (p. 336)
split peas

Beans, Canned:
black beans
garbanzo beans
kidney beans (no salt
  added)
vegetarian beans in tomato
  sauce (e.g. Heinz)

Nuts:
almonds (not roasted,
  unsalted)
*cashews (roasted, unsalted)
pecans (p. 374 only)
walnuts

Dried Fruits:
*coconut, unsweetened
dates or *date dices or
  nuggets
figs, black, Mission (p. 360
  only)
raisins

Frozen Foods:
berries (p. 367 only)
corn
green beans
peas
orange juice concentrate

Canned Food Items:
chilies, diced
fruits, unsweetened (p. 367
  only)
onion, dry minced

Newman's Own Olive Oil &
  Vinegar Dressing
pineapple, chunks,
  unsweetened
pineapple, crushed,
  unsweetened
pineapple juice,
  unsweetened
tomatoes, pieces or whole
tomato sauce
tomatoes, stewed
tuna fish, water-pack (50%
  less salt)
water chestnuts

Cooking Supplies:
apple cider vinegar
*arrowroot powder
*baking powder, low-sodium
  or Rumford
*barbecue sauce (e.g.
  Robbie's)
*Bragg Liquid Aminos
*buttermilk, powdered (e.g.
  Darigold)
canola oil (*Spectrum
  Naturals, Arrowhead
  Mills)
*carob chips, unsweetened
  (e.g. Sunspire)
catsup, no salt added (e.g.
  Featherweight**)
*chicken and/or beef broth
  (e.g. Hain or Health
  Valley)
cornstarch
*crystalline fructose
dill pickles, no salt added
  (e.g. Featherweight**)
garlic cloves

gelatin, unflavored (e.g. Knox)
honey or *unheated honey
lemon juice
*liquid lecithin (p. 371 only)
mayonnaise (e.g. Hollywood or *Hain)
mustard, no salt added (e.g. Featherweight** or *stoneground mustard)
*noninstant nonfat dry milk
olive oil or *extra virgin organic (e.g. Spectrum Naturals, Arrowhead Mills, Omega Nutrition; see also pp. 304-05)
pimiento
ripe olives, sliced (p. 334 only)
ripe olives, whole (p. 349 only)
salsa
*sea salt (e.g. RealSalt, see p. 304 to mail order)
soy sauce (e.g. Kikkoman Lite)
*Sucanat (whole cane sugar, p. 369 only)
*sweet pickle relish
tofu, long-term storage package (e.g. Mori Nu)
vanilla extract

Herbs and Spices:
basil leaves
bay leaves
cayenne (red) pepper
chili powder
cinnamon
cumin, ground seed
curry powder
dill weed
garlic powder
ginger, ground
Italian seasoning
marjoram leaves
nutmeg
onion powder
oregano leaves
parsley, dried (optional)
paprika
rosemary leaves
sage
*Spike Seasoning
tarragon (optional, p. 371 only)
thyme leaves
tumeric

Special Order:
Sue's "Kitchen Magic" Seasoning (see p. 383)

** Featherweight brand is available in several supermarkets, but not all; check also at health-food stores.

55

The Health-Food Store

———— ♥ ————

You will find many additional food items in health-food stores that are not available or are more expensive in supermarkets. Begin to investigate the resources. Take the Survey Checklist (pp. 272-75) with you. This also makes an excellent field trip for children ages 8 and older.

Supermarkets are most deficient in whole-grain flours, pastas, breads, and quality oils. The following items are a basic beginner list to stock your pantry:

whole-grain breads (as freezer space allows):
    bread for sandwiches
    dinner rolls
    hamburger buns
    tortillas, corn and whole-wheat

whole-grain pastas (freeze if unused for over 1 month):
    spaghetti, noodles, lasagna noodles

whole grains and flours:
    millet
    oat bran (keep in refrigerator or freezer)
    stoneground cornmeal
    whole-wheat pastry flour or grain
    wheat bran (keep in freezer)

oils: Spectrum Naturals, Arrowhead Mills, or Omega Nutrition
    extra virgin organic olive oil
    pure pressed or organic canola oil
    organic safflower oil, unrefined or expeller pressed

low sodium or Rumford baking powder

sea salt (RealSalt recommended; see p. 304 to mail order)

chicken and/or beef broth, salted or unsalted (Hain or Health Valley)

alfalfa seeds (for sprouts—see p. 153)

Spike—seasoning

other items needed for specific recipes within the next month

SURVEY CHECKLIST FOR THE
HEALTH-FOOD STORE

(Make several copies of this list. Visit more than one store. You'll soon know what is available and where to shop.)

Whole Grains: ___wheat ___pastry wheat
___rolled oats ___oat groats ___millet ___Kamut
___buckwheat ___triticale ___rye ___spelt
___amaranth ___short-grain brown rice ___corn
___long-grain brown rice ___basmati rice ___wild rice
___quick brown rice ___quinoa ___barley
___bulk buying option? ___organic

Whole-Grain Flours: ___winter wheat (bread flour)
___pastry flour ___oat flour ___millet flour
___buckwheat flour ___triticale flour ___amaranth flour
___cornmeal ___brown rice flour ___wheat bran
___oat bran ___Kamut flour ___spelt flour

Whole-Grain Cereals (list 4 you would like to try):

_____

_____

Whole-Grain Pastas: ___spaghetti ___macaroni
___noodles ___lasagna

Whole-Grain Crackers and Chips: ___whole wheat
___rye ___brown rice cakes ___grahams
___stoneground corn chips ___blue corn chips

Whole-Grain Breads: ___sandwich bread ___pita breads
___English muffins ___hot dog buns
___hamburger buns ___dinner rolls ___French rolls
___whole-wheat tortillas ___bagels
___stoneground corn tortillas or chapatis

Whole-Grain Mixes: ___cake ___muffin ___nut bread
___pancake ___cookie

Beans: ___ soybeans ___ lima beans ___ kidney beans
___black (turtle) beans ___pinto beans
___garbanzo beans ___ black-eyed peas___mung beans
___azuki beans ___split peas ___lentils
___red beans ___navy beans ___great northern beans
___bulk buying option? ___organic

Nuts: ___almonds ___pecans ___cashews ___walnuts
___peanuts ___pine nuts

Seeds: ___sesame ___sunflower ___pumpkin ___alfalfa
___poppy ___flax

Spreads: ___peanut butter (salt only)
___peanut butter (no salt) ___almond butter
___tahini (sesame) spread ___cashew butter
___jam (honey or unsweetened) ___pure maple syrup

Baking Items: ___low-sodium or Rumford baking powder
___sea salt ___nonfat dry milk powder ___low-fat cocoa
___carob powder ___unsweetened coconut
___roasted carob powder ___arrowroot ___carob chips
___organic extra virgin olive oil
___canola oil ___blackstrap molasses
___honey (unheated, unfiltered) ___honey ___sea salt
___crystalline fructose ___date sugar ___Sucanat
___liquid lecithin (to grease pans)
___buttermilk powder

Condiments and Cooking: ___apple cider vinegar
___soy sauce ___mayonnaise ___catsup
___pickle relish (honey-sweetened or unsweetened)
___salsa ___mustard ___salad dressings
___salad dressing mixes ___barbecue sauce
___Bragg Liquid Aminos

Dried Fruits: ___raisins ___date dices or nuggets
___apricots ___apples ___pineapple ___figs

Beverages: ___herb teas ___coffee substitutes
___natural sodas ___mineral water
___fruit juices, bottled ___fresh juices
___Swiss process decaffeinated coffee
___bottled juices (unsweetened)
___fresh vegetable juices (refrigerator)

Canned Goods: ___spaghetti or pasta sauce
___chicken broth ___beef broth ___soups
___chili con carne ___vegetarian chili

Spices and Seasonings: ___Spike

Meats, Poultry (organic or without chemicals): ___beef
___chicken ___turkey ___ground turkey

Packaged Meats (without nitrates, nitrites, or sugar):
___chicken weiners ___turkey weiners
___luncheon meat

Dairy: ___nonfat yogurt ___low-fat yogurt
___buttermilk ___goat's milk ___kefir
___raw certified milk ___raw certified whipping cream
___tofu ___kefir cheese ___low-sodium cheddar cheese
___raw certified cheese ___goat cheese
___raw certified butter ___honey ice cream
___frozen yogurt ___fertile eggs
___tofu sandwich spread

Dairy Alternatives: ___soy milk ___rice milk ___nut milks

Frozen Foods (of interest to you): ___vegetables ___fish
___prepared entrées

Fresh Produce: ___organically grown? ___large selection
___small selection

Food Supplements: ___wall-to-wall? ___bee pollen
___brewer's yeast ___psyllium seed

Health Bonuses: ___flaxseed oil ___granular lecithin
___liquid lecithin ___brewer's yeast
___fruit/vegetable cleaner

Books/Publications: ___small selection ___broad selection
___New Age influence?

56

Dining Out

———— ♥ ————

*H*ow can I continue my *Eating Better Lifestyle* when I eat out? The first step is to develop this mentality: "I am in control." You do not need to be a victim of food fare in public places! Sometimes the whole-food offerings are few, but with a little forethought and discipline you can plan your strategy. How do you evaluate food quality? The answer to that question is to define the *Eating Better Lifestyle* and look for those characteristics in public eating places.

High Fiber

Salad bars with a wide variety of fresh vegetables; some include fruits as well; look for the dark leafy greens among the iceberg lettuce. The FDA has banned sulfites to preserve freshness of salad ingredients, but ask about it anyway. Public places do not always adhere to new rulings right away.

Make the salad bar your main dish. Sunflower seeds, alfalfa sprouts, cottage cheese (low-fat, when possible), grated Parmesan cheese, and kidney and garbanzo beans can be added for protein.

Main-dish salads such as chef's, tuna, chicken, vegetarian, or taco. You can request ingredients to be left out or exchanged. For example, ham can be omitted from a chef's salad. Water-packed tuna can be used in the tuna salad. Chicken is often an option in a taco salad, and you can ask for less meat in it and more of the garden ingredients with a reduced supply of the chips.

Fresh fruit-in-season salads—plain or with plain yogurt or low-fat cottage cheese or a bit of cheddar cheese.

Whole-grain bread. Public eating places are most deficient in whole-grain breads. Whole-wheat sandwich bread is often available, but may not be entirely whole grain. Choose sourdough over others. Sourdough is usually easier to digest.

Chili and refried beans are good sources of fiber, but may be high in fat and too salty. Inquire. Request a sample. You can judge the fat and salt for yourself that way.

Save pasta dishes for home cooking when you can use whole-grain pasta. When you have a choice between rice pilaf, baked potato, or mashed potatoes, take the baked potato. The rice is white and the mashed potatoes usually are from a box of potato flakes.

Baked potato makes a good main dish. Learn to enjoy the skin! With a salad the baked potato can be a satisfying and totally nutritious main dish. It is not fattening and provides good protein (see below).

Low Fat

Topping for the baked potato: You can complement the protein by requesting a protein topping instead of the usual butter or margarine. Ask the waitress to give half sour cream blended with half low-fat cottage cheese or plain yogurt. Or you can take your little container of nonfat or low-fat yogurt from home and mix it with the sour cream. Put plenty on the potato to provide that pleasing contrast in hot and cold temperature and to moisten the potato so it isn't dry. A $1/4$-cup blend of low-fat yogurt and sour cream will provide 111 calories, 5.5 grams protein, and 8 grams fat. If you use low-fat cottage cheese in place of the sour cream you will have 95 calories, 10.5 grams of protein, and only 2.5 grams of fat! Quite an improvement over even one tablespoon of butter at 102 calories, with no protein and 12 grams of fat.

At the salad bar, leave the prepared salads such as macaroni, potato, and coleslaw with lots of mayonnaise in them behind. Three-bean salad, well-drained, or pickled vegetables add tang without the fat.

Choose lemon juice, vinegar and olive oil, or cottage cheese as good salad toppings in place of oil dressings. If you use oil dressing, aim for one tablespoon well-distributed over the greenery.

Request salad dressings, gravies, and sauces to be served on the side. Let 1 tablespoon be your measuring guide.

Order meats that are baked or broiled, and unbreaded. Choose fish and chicken instead of beef. Request fish to be cooked without fat. Remove the skin from the chicken. Roast beef has less fat than hamburger.

If you don't order refined-white-flour rolls or bread, you won't have a decision to make about using butter on them.

Ask for butter in place of margarine. This goes against what everyone else says to do (see pp. 107-08). Limit yourself to one pat.

Main dishes with cheese sauce or cream sauce will be very high in fat. If you want one of these, order one dish for two people, eat a small portion, and fill up on fresh salad.

Skip cakes, pies, quick breads, cream cheese, and ice cream desserts. Have fresh fruit, frozen yogurt, or a taste of someone else's dessert.

For children order water, real fruit juice, or nonfat milk to drink. Most children enjoy orange juice. Avoid homogenized milk (see pp. 126-27).

Avoid deep-fat-fried foods such as French fries, fried chicken, fried shrimp, and scallops. You can take the skin off fried chicken, however.

If you order a vegetarian hot dish, request that only a very small amount of fat, such as in stir-fry, be used. Some places use a lot!

Choose clear soups with vegetables, chicken, or beef in preference to cream soups. Find out, however, if a lot of fat is in the broth and request "not salty." Ask for a taste first! Ask if it is homemade. They are usually better.

Not Too Much

This is more a matter of discipline and self-control. Some commitments made in advance will help. First, decide not to order a full dinner per person. Order salad or soup for each person and share a dinner between two people. Practically every restaurant dinner is big enough for two!

Tortilla chip appetizer in Mexican restaurants: Make a prior commitment to let the first bowlful suffice. If you like the appetizer "hot," order extra salsa and enjoy much "hot" with few chips.

Order soup and salad and nothing else. Wait until you have finished before ordering anything more. You probably won't want anything else!

Less Salt

Leave the salt shaker in its place on the table.

Request that meats, fish, poultry be cooked without salt.

Ask to taste the soup before ordering. Oversalting soups is a common practice. If enough customers ask about this, chefs will catch on.

Skip potato chips, French fries, breaded meats, and breaded fish.

Casserole dishes will be higher in salt than fresh salads and fruits.

Low Sweets

Order fresh fruit or frozen yogurt for dessert.

Skip dessert or have a taste of someone else's.

Don't order muffins, nut breads, cornbread, or quick breads, in general. These have more sugar in them than yeast breads such as dinner rolls, sandwich breads, and crusty French loaves. Almost all of them are made with white flour, anyway.

Natural-Food Restaurants

Now you have the general guidelines. What are the best restaurants to look for? Natural-food restaurants have much more to offer nutritionally than other restaurants. Usually you will have a good variety of whole-grain breads, brown rice, and whole-grain pasta dishes to choose from. There is more variety in the salad greenery and more opportunity to find dishes utilizing meats in smaller quantity. Sometimes vegetable oil can be overused. It is a good idea to ask about the amount used. Natural-food restaurants offer greater variety of imaginative dishes utilizing fresh vegetables and fruits. Some vegetarian restaurants have an Eastern cultic atmosphere. If you take guests to one of these, make sure they will not feel uncomfortable there.

Ethnic Food

Ethnic foods often offer more nutrition than traditional American fare. Chinese restaurants offer more vegetables.

You can ask for the MSG (monosodium glutamate) to be omitted. Oriental restaurants seldom serve brown rice. If you like Chinese food, ask for brown rice. If proprietors hear such requests from customers repeatedly, they will begin to catch on. Businesses want to please their customers. Repeat business means profit.

Many Japanese restaurants offer both plant and fish seafood, tofu, and many vegetables. Avoid the deep-fried foods, especially the shellfish. Sushi (raw fish wrapped in a variety of ingredients) is usually safe to eat.

Indian restaurants are not common, but Indian food offers some good choices, such as curry dishes and yogurt. Mexican food can be a better choice than standard American fast foods. Request corn tortillas that are not fried. They can be warmed without fat. Choose the dishes with lots of greenery. Most Mexican food has more greenery and beans and less meat. The beans may contain lard, however. Go for the salad-type dishes in preference to ones with cheese.

What About Fast Foods?

Drive by them fast! The problem is not the "fast" but the food. Look for what isn't fried, what isn't refined, what isn't oversalted, and what isn't full of sugar. Some fast-food places are installing salad bars. Opt for the pizza parlor ahead of the hamburger, fried chicken, or fish 'n' chips places. Although pizza is made with a white flour crust, there is a higher proportion of nonmeat goodies on top. Skip the pepperoni and try for plain cheese or the vegetable-topped choices. Order a small serving of pizza and take a big salad with it. Actually, if you really want a hamburger and have access to a natural-foods restaurant, buy a hamburger there on a whole-wheat bun with extra fresh ingredients.

Traveling by Air?

You can request three days ahead for special meals on most airlines. Your travel agent can also do this for you.

Emilie does this often. She has received beautiful salads, vegetable meals, pasta, and fruit platters. Remember that good business is serving the customer's wishes!

Traveling by Car?

As long-distance travelers, Rich and Sue have developed a system for eating out that is enjoyable and uncomplicated. They carry granola and buy fresh fruit, yogurt, and skim milk along the way for breakfasts. For lunches they buy leafy lettuce, a tomato, cheddar cheese, Hollywood mayonnaise, carrots, a couple pieces of fresh fruit, and real fruit juice. At a rest stop they prepare a vegetable salad or sandwiches (if whole-wheat bread is available). For dinner they eat out following the guidelines we've listed. The food expense is very low. Eating out costs twice as much as eating the same meal at home.

When Rich and Sue traveled to Mexico City by train, granola, yogurt, fresh fruit purchased along the way, and their own water supply were sustaining and satisfying.

Eating with Friends

It won't be long before your friends realize that you like healthy food. In the meantime, offer to bring one of the dishes. You can't go wrong by offering to bring the salad, some muffins, or the dessert. This gives you the opportunity to introduce whole foods in a winsome way. You don't have to make any comments about what you bring or what you are served. Eat smaller amounts of the less-nutritious items and larger amounts of the more-nutritious. Thank your host and hostess for their hospitality. Don't discuss nutrition unless you are invited to answer some questions or inquiries.

If you know your conscience will bother you if you eat a certain food such as pork, let your hostess know in advance that you do not eat that food. This need not be offensive. What is offensive is passing judgment, showing disdain, or rejecting food when it is set in front of you. If you have a health problem such as allergies, your hostess will be only too glad to omit it from the menu if you inform her in advance.

Potlucks and Smorgasbords

These occasions are temptations to gorge, so you'll need to exercise a little restraint. Usually there is a wide enough variety to find some nutritious selections. Sue always takes a big fresh salad and whole-grain muffins or rolls so that there are at least two nutritious items. Eating at a potluck is not the same as eating with friends in their home. People usually don't pay much attention to whose dishes you eat or what you eat at a potluck.

Breakfast Out?

Fresh fruit, real fruit juice, hot or cold cereal, whole-wheat toast with butter and/or honey, decaffeinated coffee or tea, and egg omelets that aren't too cheesy, or poached eggs are good choices. Avoid the pancakes, waffles, French toast, and muffins unless they are whole-grain. Omit the bacon and pork sausage. If you desire meat, ask for a small lean beef patty in place of the pork. If you like potatoes, request that they be fried in one tablespoon or less of fat.

A Few Extras

Peppermint or spearmint tea sipped slowly with the meal will assist in digestion of the food. Take your own tea bags and ask for hot water.

Meats eaten after salads may hinder digestion. Eat the meat with the salad.

Let the establishment know that you appreciate choices. Some restaurants request written evaluations. Be sure to write on it that you would like the option to order whole-grain bread or rolls and brown rice.

In lieu of sour cream request a blend of sour cream and nonfat or low-fat yogurt. Again, if proprietors get requests often enough, they will begin to oblige. Tradition fogs imagination. Some things, such as keeping yogurt on hand, would be such an easy thing to do.

Request purified or bottled water. You can also request fresh lemon to squeeze into it.

Remember, you are in control! Ask for exactly what you want even if you know the establishment doesn't have it. Consumer demand is what elicits change in our profit-oriented society.

57

Food Storage and Safety Tips

———— ♥ ————

♥ Make sure your refrigerator is 40° or less and your freezer 0° or less.

♥ After opening, refrigerate wheat germ, pure maple syrup, vegetable oils, salad dressings, mayonnaise, jams, jellies, peanut butter without sugar or hydrogenated fat added, and shelled nuts.

♥ Store shelled nuts, sunflower seeds, and sesame seeds purchased in quantity in the freezer.

♥ Uncooked bulgur (parboiled wheat) does not require refrigeration even during the hot days of summer. Neither does white rice. Brown rice also keeps well unrefrigerated for a month, and refrigerated for six months.

♥ When you store basic ingredients such as canned broth or tomatoes, rotate the older containers to the front of your cupboard or refrigerator or date them with a marking pen to use first.

- ♥ To prevent contamination of food inside containers, always use a clean utensil to scoop out mayonnaise, peanut butter, tomato paste, etc. Never eat directly from the container except for one taste with a clean utensil.

- ♥ To reduce contact with air which may cause food to deteriorate more quickly, store foods and leftovers in the smallest possible containers. This also gives you more room in the refrigerator.

- ♥ In warm weather, unless your kitchen is air-conditioned, consider storing whole-grain flours, crackers, and breads in the refrigerator or freezer, unless you can use them quickly. Refrigeration tends to dry out breads. Slice loaves first and freeze them unless they are to be eaten within three or four days.

- ♥ Whole-grain crackers with no preservatives added go rancid quickly. Store in refrigerator or freezer if not used up in a couple of weeks.

- ♥ To keep crackers crisp, store them in a canister with a dry paper towel inside the cover. To recrisp soft crackers, place them on a cookie sheet in a 250° oven for about 10 minutes.

- ♥ Honey keeps best in a warm, dark place. It will crystallize in the refrigerator making it inconvenient to use. Warm crystallized honey over low heat in a pan of water to reliquefy it.

- ♥ We love raisins that are soft and chewy in cereal. Buy cold cereals plain and a large package of raisins. Pour 1/2 cup boiling water over the raisins in a jar, cover tightly with a lid and shake up a bit. Let cool and refrigerate until cereal time. Take out as many as needed.

- ♥ When using a grater, put masking tape or a bandage on your thumb. It works every time—and no more hurt thumb.

- ♥ Frozen foods have a definite freezer life. Use food within the specified period of time. Meats, such as ground beef, turkey, and franks keep 2–3 months, roast beef up to 12 months. Wrap properly in freezer wrap. Wax paper won't do. Sandwich meats keep only one month. Mark packages with "USE BY" date. Your market does this, and it makes good sense.

♥ To clean and store fresh produce to preserve freshness and nutrients, see chapters 25 and 27.

Useful Leftovers

♥ Chop small amounts of leftover cooked turkey, chicken, or beef into chunks for adding to soup, a hearty main dish, chili, or spaghetti.

♥ Freeze the few extra tablespoons of fruit juice left in the bottom of the container in an ice cube tray. Pop the cubes into a plastic bag to store until you roast a turkey or chicken. Perfect for basting!

♥ Put leftover rice in a greased casserole and cover with homemade cheese sauce. Sprinkle with grated cheese and bake at 350° for 20 minutes, or use leftover rice in stuffing as a substitute for bread. Also great for putting into soups or making rice pudding.

♥ Save leftover pancakes or waffles. Pop them into the toaster or oven for a quick, easy breakfast or after-school snack. Waffles also reheat perfectly in the waffle iron set at medium temperature.

♥ Keep a leftover list on the refrigerator with date stored and what container item is stored in. Write item on menu where you can use it up.

Time-Saver Tips

♥ Make your own convenience foods. Chop large batches of onion, green pepper, or nuts and freeze in small units. Grate a week's or month's worth of cheese and freeze it in recipe-size portions. Shape ground meat or ground turkey into patties so you can thaw a few at a time. Freeze homemade casseroles, soups, stews, and chili in serving-size portions for faster thawing and reheating. Meal planning will help you take advantage of doing these things!

♥ Leave bread "rejects" in a basket to dry in the open air. When you have several slices, make crumbs with them in the blender and freeze in a tightly covered Tupperware container or a plastic bag. They'll be ready to use when you need them.

♥ To speed up baking potatoes, put a clean nail through the potato and it will bake in half the time.

♥ For quick, easy cleanup when preparing sticky hot cereal or steaming rice, coat the inside of the saucepan with vegetable cooking spray beforehand. Try it also on the blades of the food processor when mixing dough.

♥ When measuring oil and honey, measure the oil before the honey. The honey will pour right out of the oiled measuring cup.

♥ Keep a grocery list on your refrigerator or bulletin board and write down each item when you notice that you need to restock. By the time you are ready to shop, all the "extras" that you might otherwise forget are already listed.

♥ Make cleanup after each food preparation part of the preparation. Clutter from the last task will not be in your way and by mealtime your kitchen will be clean.

♥ For baking projects such as muffins, set out and measure ingredients, chop nuts, etc. earlier in the day. Leave only mixing and baking for the last minute. Assemble casseroles at a more leisurely hour. See also, "What About Time?" chapter 12.

Utensils and Equipment for the Kitchen

Here is a list of basics you should have when cooking:

Liquid measuring cups—2-cup measure will handle many jobs.

Dry measuring cups—These usually come in nested sets from 1/4 to 1 cup.

Measuring spoons—These also come in sets which include 1/4 teaspoon, 1/2 teaspoon, 1 teaspoon, and 1 tablespoon.

Wooden spoons and large metal spoons—A cook should have several of each kind. A slotted spoon is also useful.

Rubber spatulas—You should have at least one wide one; a narrow rubber spatula is useful for scraping out jars and small bowls.

All-purpose scoop—Dispenses cookie dough like a larger one dispenses ice cream. Handy for all kinds of cookie doughs—stiff or soupy! Great for meatballs, too. Usually available at kitchen specialty shops. Get the 1″ size.

Lemon zester—To grate lemon or orange peel, this is much easier than using the fine grater holes of a shredder.

Wire whisk—A wire whisk at least as long as a rubber scraper will perform many important hand-blending jobs. A mini-sized whisk is helpful for small amounts, such as blending salad dressing.

Oven thermometer—Essential for gauging accurate temperature for most ovens. Purchase at supermarket.

Mixing bowl set—Set of three: small, medium, large; Pyrex or stainless steel.

Crockpot—Great time-saver for cooking dry beans, chicken with broth, stews, soups.

Frying pan—A large frying pan with a lid is used in many different kinds of recipes. We recommend stainless steel as the safest material for most cooking over direct heat.

Omelet pan—A 7″-8″ fry pan with curved sides. We recommend stainless steel, well seasoned (see *Eating Better Breakfasts*, p. 384, for purchasing and seasoning an omelet pan).

Griddle—There is nothing like a cast-iron griddle for pancakes, if you can find one (we found one in a specialty shop in Port Gamble, WA). To season a new griddle, wash it with warm water and dry well. Put over a very hot burner, add a few tablespoons olive or peanut oil, and swirl it around the pan. Pour off the oil, cool the pan, and repeat the process. Food will not stick to a properly seasoned pan.

Waffle iron—You won't want to miss our fantastic wholegrain *5-Minute Blender Waffles* (see recipe section)! We recommend using small waffle irons. Most are nonstick.

Baking pans—Stainless steel or Pyrex. Include an 8″ or 9″ square pan, two or three 9″ round cake pans, 9″ x 13″ pan, 8½″ x 4½″ loaf pan (medium size), angel food cake tube pan, bundt cake pan, 9½″ pie pan, muffin pan with 1¼″ deep cups (the deeper size), and one or two cookie sheets.

Knives—A good knife is worth its weight in gold. It can make cooking tasks so much easier. We recommend a good paring knife, a French chef's knife, a curved boning knife, and a serrated bread knife. A chef's knife makes wonderfully light work of chopping nuts, dried fruits, apples, and vegetables, and shredding cabbage. A curved boning knife is just right for curved fruits and slicing. We think the best way to purchase these is not in a fancy department store set, but individually at a restaurant supply store with a knowledgeable clerk's help.

Whetstone—Make lighter work of chopping and cutting by keeping your knives sharp! Purchase this at a hardware store. It will last for your lifetime and probably your grandchildren's. Forget the electric knife sharpener and the longhandled round knife sharpener.

Blender—Indispensable to whole food preparation and a "must" for our blender batter baking that you won't want to miss (see *5-Minute Blender Waffles & Pancakes* in recipe section). One that will crack ice, make bread crumbs, chop nuts, and mince parsley will do almost anything else you'll need, plus blend waffles and pancakes. A 10-speed Oster-izer, for example, works well.

Garlic press—Buy one that crushes garlic without peeling it—so easy! Available in kitchen specialty shops. Make sure it is very strong (many garlic presses are real "duds").

Shredder—One with fine holes for grating things such as lemon peel; another with larger holes for grating cheese, cabbage, and carrots.

Timer—Most stoves have timers, but if yours does not work, there are hand-held timers that are very accurate.

Tongs—To lift things out of water.

Colander—For draining things like spaghetti.

Rolling pin—An essential if you're going to make pastry.

Saucepans—Buy the best you can afford. A good, strong pan with a riveted handle and thick bottom will last a life-time. It's nice to have a 1-quart, 2-quart, and 3-quart sauce-pan. But if you can only choose one, select a good 2-quart saucepan. Consider a stainless steel, waterless one.

Wire racks—For cooling cookies, cakes, breads.

Electric mixer—There are many different kinds. Even small, hand-held ones make cooking tasks easier.

Wok—Makes quick, light work of stir-frying, especially a nonstick electric one. Also useful for steaming large amounts of food such as big pieces of squash or pumpkin, or a large bunch of dark leafy greens.

58

How to Read a Label

————— ♥ —————

ood companies thrive on the nutritional half-truth that will sell the product. These selling points are printed in large letters on the front of the package. Do not buy a product merely because one of the following terms appears on the front: "no preservatives added," "all-natural," "100% natural," "no sugar added," "low calorie," "low fat," "fat-free," "no salt added," "low cholesterol." These facts may be important, but you'll want to know much more. For example, many products without preservatives are refined carbohydrates containing mostly white flour and white sugar. Any product can be labeled "natural" and contain white flour and white sugar since both ingredients are food. Find out all the ingredients in the product.

The Ingredients List
(the best guide to quality)

The most important part of the label is the ingredients list in fine print on the back, side, or end of the container. Ingredients are listed in descending amounts by weight. The first listed ingredient is the most by weight in the product. Watch for several different kinds of sugars listed.

If there are two or three kinds, there may be more sugar in the product than the first-named ingredient. For example: "wheat flour, brown sugar, soybean oil, honey, yeast, salt."

Ingredients to avoid are: hydrogenated fat or vegetable oil, partially hydrogenated fat or vegetable oils, shortening, refined sugars such as high fructose corn syrup, corn syrup solids, sucrose, dextrose, sugar, brown sugar, wheat flour (it is white unless designated whole wheat), enriched white or wheat flour, bleached enriched white flour, degerminated cornmeal.

There are thousands of additives, with new ones emerging daily. To know about every one is impossible. More important is that the products containing additives seldom include whole-food ingredients as the primary ingredients. If the product does not contain real whole-food ingredients, it isn't nutritionally worth buying anyway. Check the top ten additives to avoid, p. 188. The cumulative effects of preservatives on the human body are not known. Although you should read labels in every store, you will have a much easier time finding prepackaged convenience foods without additives in health-food stores. A "must" reference to additives is *A Consumer's Dictionary of Food Additives* (see Recommended Reading, p. 379).

Nutrient Data and the New Labeling Law

The 1990 Nutrition Labeling and Education Act has mandated standardized nutrition labeling on all packaged foods. This is a revolution in food package labeling! By May 1994, 70% of all processed foods already carried the new label. All package labels must carry the same strict format with the same nutrient information. Once you understand how to recognize, read, and use this label you can apply your knowledge to every product. That's the good part.

Study the standardized nutrition label on p. 294.

Everything on it is now required by law. Note the *7 parts*. This will be a writing exercise, so get out your pencil and fill in the blanks on pages 295-96 (using the information on the sample label).

1. NATURAL GRANOLA

NUTRITION FACTS

2. Serving Size 2/3 cup (55g)
Servings per Container 8

3. **Amount per Serving**

Calories 230   Calories from Fat 50

% Daily Value*

4.

Total Fat 6g	**9%**
Saturated Fat 1g	**5%**
Cholesterol 0mg	**0%**
Sodium 20mg	**1%**
Total Carbohydrate 40g	**13%**
Dietary Fiber 4g	**16%**
Sugars 13g	
Protein 7g	

5.

Vitamin A 0%	•	Vitamin C 0%
Calcium 0%	•	Iron 6%

6. * Percent Daily Values are based on a 2,000 calorie diet.
Your daily values may be higher or lower depending
on your calorie needs:

	Calories	2,000	2,500
Total Fat	Less than	65g	80g
Sat Fat	Less than	20g	25g
Cholesterol	Less than	300mg	300mg
Sodium	Less than	2,400mg	2,400mg
Total carbohydrate		300g	375g
Dietary Fiber		25g	30g

7. Calories per gram:
Fat 9   •   Carbohydrates 4   •   Protein 4

That was the easy part. Now for the interpretation. I
hope you will endure through this because there is a valuable lesson in it.

We are going to take a glimpse into the minds of nutritional technocrats. If it sounds complicated, that's okay—read through to the end anyway.

1. The name of the product _____

2. Serving Size _____

3. Amount per Serving:
   Calories _____ Calories from Fat _____

4.

	Number of grams	% Daily Value*
Total Fat		
Saturated Fat		
Cholesterol		
Sodium		
Total Carbohydrate		
Dietary Fiber		
Sugars		
Protein		

5. Percentage of the RDA (Recommended Daily Allowances) of selected nutrients (Vitamins A and C, Calcium, Iron)

   Vitamin A _____ Vitamin C _____
   Calcium_____Iron _____

6. *Definition of *Daily Value*, followed by a list of daily values in grams not to be exceeded for a healthy diet (don't list the values; just write out the definition of *Daily Value*):

   _____

   _____

   _____

7. Calories per 1 gram of fat, carbohydrate, protein:

Fat _____   Carbohydrate _____   Protein _____

The key to making sense of the label is to clearly understand what *Daily Value* is. *Daily Value is the daily intake or
amount of grams or milligrams of each selected nutrient that you
should not exceed daily, based on your total calorie intake of food.*
Since calorie intake varies for everyone, the standardized
label obviously focuses on a common average (*2000 calories—
an average for most women, and 2500 calories—an average for
most men.* Note those amounts in part 6 of the label).

Assume for now that you consume 2000 calories daily.
Based on this calorie intake, note the amounts of the specified nutrients you should consume listed in part 6: less
than 65 g (grams) of fat, less than 20 grams saturated fat,
less than 300 mg. cholesterol, less than 2400 mg. sodium, a
total of 300 grams carbohydrate, and 25 grams dietary
fiber. *These are your Daily Values.*

Now return to part 4 of the label. What is the % Daily
Value listed for *Total Fat?* It is 9%. But 9% of *what?* This is the
KEY to understanding what the label means. To answer this
question, look in part 6 again to see what your limit of Total
Fat grams should be on a 2000-calorie diet. It is less than 65
grams fat (practically speaking, just 65 grams). Now return
to part 4 of the label and note how many grams of *Total Fat*
are in one serving of the product. The total is 6 grams. The
6 grams of Total Fat in this product is *9% of your limit of 65
grams fat per day (your Daily Value for fat).* Let's check this out.
Get out your calculator. Divide 6 grams by 65 grams (punch
6 on your calculator, punch the division sign, punch 65,
press the equal sign). You should get 0.0923076. Round it
off to .09 (9%). It helps to visualize this as a fraction $^6/_{65}$ =
.09 = 9%.

One serving of this product (Natural Granola) provides
you with 9% of the 65 grams of total fat you should limit
yourself to for one day. How many servings of Natural
Granola would you need to eat to hit 100% of your Daily

Value for fat (a total of 65 grams)? You would need to divide 100% by 9%. Do it on your calculator. Your answer should be 11.111111. Round it off to 11—11 *what?*—11 servings of Natural Granola. Now multiply 6 grams by 11 servings (6 x 11 = 66 grams fat—that's close enough!). *Whew!* Were you ready for this? You don't have to check out the figures on the label, of course, in order to use them. But if you don't understand how the nutritional technocrats arrived at that 9%, you will continue to be confused about what "Daily Value" means. Return to part 6. There are five more percentages listed. Check each one of them out with your calculator the same way we did for the Total Fat. Did you find that they were correct? I guarantee that if you can readily do this calculation with understanding, you will know what the percentages are based on: *the number of grams or milligrams of each selected nutrient that you should not exceed daily, based on your total calorie intake of food—that is, the Daily Value.* Note that the Daily Values for total carbohydrate and total dietary fiber are not daily limits but reasonable amounts for a 2000-calorie diet.

Now let's try to apply this information to reality to decide if it is an important part of "a realistic approach to a healthy lifestyle." We'll just stick with the fat, though. Your goal is to eat 65 grams or less for the day. How will you keep track of the percent of fat you've eaten if you don't add the percentages up? That is the only way you will know when you've reached 100%. So you ate one serving of five different packaged foods. One serving of one food gave you 9% fat, another 15%, a third 6%, another 20%, and finally the fifth 16%. Add them up: 9 + 15 + 6 + 20 + 16 = 66%. You've now eaten 66% percent of your Daily Value of fat (65 grams). You can have 34% more fat for the day (34% of your "Daily Value," that is—you must keep reminding yourself of this until you have it memorized). What's on the rest of the menu for the day? Let's say this includes your favorite waffle recipe for breakfast, a homemade shake and an apple for lunch, and a main dish recipe you prepared for dinner, plus a lovely tossed salad. *Now what?* These food items don't come ready-made with Nutrition Facts labels! But don't worry. The nutritional technocrats have probably already recognized this problem and are diligently working on nutrient tables you can get from books for all those other foods you ate that didn't come in a package. It was tedious enough having to add up five things you ate out of packages! Don't even think about what it would be like to add up the percentages of six to ten ingredients you used in a recipe!

There must be a better way. Busy women don't have time to punch calculators all day. After having done so, they still wouldn't have the necessary information for about half the foods they eat, anyway—at least not without reading a book! Just how did the technocrats decide that if I eat 2000 calories in a day (which I may or may not) I should limit my "Daily Value" of fat to 65 grams? Here is the answer. The USDA has determined that our fat intake should not exceed 25% to 30% of our total calories. If you multiply 65 grams of fat by 9 (because there are 9 calories in each gram of fat; part 7 on our sample label, p. 294) you will get 585 ($65 \times 9 = 585$ calories). Thus 65 grams of fat = 585 calories of fat. Divide 585 calories by 2000 calories on your calculator (punch in 585, punch the divide sign, punch in 2000, punch the equal sign). The answer should be 0.2925. Round it off to 0.29 (29%). Again it helps to understand this by visualizing it as a fraction: $585/2000 = 0.29$ (29%).

Thus, 585 calories of fat = 29% of 2000 calories, within the 25% to 30% recommended limit of total fat.

Isn't there a simpler way to watch fat intake? Here is one way you might do it. See if it sounds easier: You know that your daily fat limit should be 65 grams because that amount is 29% of your 2000-calorie daily intake of food (that is, if you eat 2000 calories—are you prepared to count those, too?). Why not just add up the number of fat grams in each serving of each packaged food you eat in a day? If you are using our recipes, you could add the grams of those in, too.

You could put a chart of the number of fat grams of other common foods that don't have labels on them on your refrigerator so you could add them in, also. But you are still "counting." I predict that would last about one to three days.

Let's try another method: Suppose that our Natural Granola Nutrition Facts label listed the percentage of calories that come from fat in one serving? Suppose it was 21%. It you ate a serving of the granola, what percent of fat did you eat? Twenty-one percent of course. Is that within the recommended daily limit? Yes, because the recommended limit is 25% to 30% of calories. Let's say you eat one serving of each of five different packaged foods. Each package states what percent of the calories is fat in a serving. Suppose they are 15%, 30%, 25%, 8%, 12%. Would you have to add them up? Would you have to know how many calories you actually ate? The answer to both those questions is NO. As long as you know the percentage of fat of any food is not over 30% of its own calories, you will not exceed your limit by eating it. Does this seem a little easier?

Now the information needed to determine the fat percentage of calories of the food itself is provided on the new standardized Nutrition Facts label. You can use it to good advantage, and it's quite easy to figure out. Return to part 3 of the label sample, p. 294. Note that the total calories per serving of Natural Granola is 230. Now note that the total calories from fat is 50. Divide 50 calories by 230. Visualize it in a fraction: $50/230 = 0.217$ (21%).

You don't need to read any further than part 3 on the label, divide the calories from fat by the total calories per serving which will give you the percentage of the calories of fat. And if it is 30% or less, you stayed within your limit. Do the same thing with the next item you eat—no adding percentages together is needed. But *wait*. What if you eat a cookie that is 50% fat and an apple that is 9% fat. Do you know whether together these two add up to 30% or less fat? It is not worth the bother. Our lives are too busy for all that!

But I do want you to know something *very important:* Each of our recipes and menus in the recipe section of this book and in the *Eating Better Cookbooks* includes the percentage of fat *based on the total calories of that recipe or menu* and *not* on the Daily Values listed on the new standardized labels of packaged foods. Turn, for example, to p. 337. Note the Menu Suggestion for *Creamy Vegetable Chowder*. What is the total percentage of fat? It is 15%. This means that 15% of the total calories for that menu is fat. That is, the fat is 15% of 587 calories. So you eat the 587 calories and get 15% worth of fat calories. Is that within the 25% to 30% recommended daily limit? Yes—in fact, it's much lower! But knowing the fat percentage of a food, recipe, or menu based on calories of that food, recipe, or menu, you know immediately if it is within the recommended limit—no adding, no dividing, no multiplying. Nobody has time to do it anyway for hundreds of recipes and menus (except Sue—and she uses a computer and data base, of course). This means you can eat delicious food without a calculator while staying within the recommended dietary limits.

Now back to the package label. If you want to know if a packaged food is a low-fat, moderate fat, or high-fat food, you need to know what percentage of its calories are fat calories. You can do that by dividing the fat calories listed in part 2 of the label by the total calories per serving listed in part 2, which we just did (see the $^{50}/_{230}$ example above). If the answer is 30% or less, classify it as low-fat. That's not the way the nutrition technocrats want you to classify it, but that's the way I recommend you classify it. It is a more realistic classification. According to the new labeling law, a packaged food cannot be labeled "low" in a nutrient unless the content per serving is 5% or less of the Daily Value. That means our Natural Granola may not legally be labeled "low-fat" because its fat content is 9% of Daily Value—well above the 5% limit. Yet only 21% of its calories come from fat—well below the recommended daily limit.

Now it's time to get realistic. Have I frustrated you with

all this technocratic jargon? As far as I am concerned, it is not far from madness. Food preparation is mainly an art. Eating is a social event. I do not think that our Lord intended us to turn food into a numbers game. We don't have time for numbers, and we don't eat numbers. We eat food that we can see, taste, smell, and feel. New standardized nutrient labeling or no nutrient labeling, the *ingredients* list on the label of any packaged food still remains the best guide to nutritional quality. Likewise, the best guide to the nutritional value of our recipes and menus is the quality of ingredients used in them. Yes, the quality is measured by the nutrients in the recipes, but you can know the quality without knowing the details of the nutrient value. Let me illustrate. For years I prepared our *Minute Bran Muffins* with better-quality ingredients than the original recipe without knowing the nutrition facts. I had no nutrient data program to calculate the information. I just knew that whole wheat had more vitamins, minerals, and fiber in it than white flour, and so on for the other ingredients. I learned general principles of quality food selection long before I began calculating grams or percentages of this and that. When I did get around to it, the nutritional quality was verified every time by the numbers. But I didn't need the numbers to make wise food choices.

So when you shop for packaged foods, you can pay a little attention to the Nutrition Facts label if you want to, but pay a lot of attention to the ingredients list. That is where nutritional quality is best evaluated. This is equally true of our recipes and menus. Even though we have provided useful nutrient data information, I intend that you treat it a little like insurance. You know it's there when you need it, but you don't pay attention to it all the time. The numbers certainly do validate the nutritional quality of the *Eating Better Lifestyle* and also assure the users of our recipes and menus that we've done our homework. So please, whatever you do with the numbers, keep it simple and enjoy the food!

A Comparison

Read the labels of the following two products. Both are the same food item. Which one would you buy—without referring to the Nutrition Facts label of either one? Do you think if you read the Nutrition Facts labels on these two different brands that they would verify that you made the better choice? I can assure you that they would! But the Nutrition Facts label can't tell you other things you need to know, such as the quality of the fat, the quality of the sugar, of the salt, of the protein, or of the carbohydrate, nor anything about the additives or preservatives. The sum of food is greater than its numbers! So give serious attention to the ingredients list and take the Nutrition Facts label with a grain of salt.

---

1 *Ingredients*: 100% whole-wheat flour, amaranth flour, pure honey, unsulphured molasses, graham flour, soybean oil, baking soda, lecithin, salt

---

2 *Ingredients*: enriched wheat flour (containing niacin, reduced iron, thiamine mononitrate and riboflavin), sugar, graham flour, partially hydrogenated vegetable shortening (contains one or more of the following: soybean oil, coconut oil, palm oil, cottonseed oil), brown sugar, corn syrup, honey, sodium bicarbonate, salt, molasses, lecithin, malted cereal syrup and vanillin

59

How to Locate Shopping Resources

———— ♥ ————

*L*ook in the Yellow Pages of your phone book under the following topics. These can lead you to other resources. Call companies on the phone and ask questions that concern you: Do you market organic or organic certified products? Do you mail order? Do you order or sell in bulk? Can you refer me to someone who sells (names of item/s)?

Bakers
Beans—Dried
Cookware
Dehydrating Equipment
Eggs
Fish
Flea Markets
Flour Dealers
Food Products
Foods, Dehydrated and Freeze-Dried
Fruits and Vegetables
Grain Dealers

Health
Herbs
Honey
Magic Mill & Mixer (look in white pages)
Meat
Milk
Nuts
Poultry
Spices
Vitamins and Food Supplements

Friends are often the best leads to unique local resources such as food co-ops, offerings of local farmers and bee-keepers, produce stands or shops, flea markets, etc.

Mail-Order Sources

Send for a catalog, price list, and shipping information from any of the sources listed below.

The Meat Shop
6522 Fremont N.
Seattle, WA 98103
(206) 783-5751
Certified organic, no hormones or antibiotics. Chickens, turkey, Shelton frozen poultry, fresh fish, beef, lamb, veal, packaged meats without nitrates or nitrites, MSG, or other preservatives.

Walnut Acres
Penns Creek, PA 17862
24-Hour credit-card line:
(717) 837-0601
Organic, chemical-free, and nonorganic. Complete line of whole-food products, family-size packages.

Mountain Ark Trading Company
120 South East Avenue
Fayettville, AR 72701
(800) 643-8909
Many organic. Complete line of staple whole-food products. Specializes in macrobiotic foods—miso, sea vegetables, etc.

Pine Ridge Farms
P.O. Box 98
Subiaco, AR 72865
(501) 934-4565
Certified organic. Chickens, turkey, ground turkey.

Oak Manor Farms
R.R. 1 Tavistock
Ontario, Canada
NOB 2R0
(519) 662-2385
Certified organic. Grains, flours, seeds, cereals, no-salt chips, pastas, nuts, dried fruits, carob chips/powder, yeast, baking powder.

American Orsa, Inc.
75 North State Street
Redmond, UT 84652
(801) 529-7487
RealSalt: unheated natural mineral salt—2, 5, 25, 50 lbs.

Giusto's Specialty Foods, Inc.
241 East Harris Avenue
South San Francisco, CA 94080
Organic. Beans, grains, flours, flakes, cereals, oils, seeds, spices, baking powder, oils, sea salt.

Deer Valley Farm
R.D. 1
Guilford, NY 13780
(607) 794-8556
Organic. Complete line of
staple whole foods. Beef,
lamb, fish, ground turkey,
Dr. Bronner's Balanced
Protein Seasoning (same as
Bernard Jensen's Natural
Vegetable Seasoning).

Arrowhead Mills, Inc.
P.O. Box 2059
Hereford, TX 79045
Organic. Grains, cereals,
flakes, beans, nuts, seeds,
dried fruits and vegetables.

Shelton Farms
204 N. Lorraine
Pomona, CA 91767
(714) 623-4361
Organic. Chickens, turkey,
ground turkey, chicken and
turkey pot pies, turkey
sausage links.

Jaffe Bros.
P.O. Box 636
Valley Center, CA 92082-0636
(619) 749-1133
Organic. Dried fruits, nuts/
butters, grains, pastas,
seeds, beans, honey, carob,
coconut, extra virgin oil,
olives, peas and beans,
mushrooms, pickles, relish.

**Flour Mills and Bread
Kneaders**
Eating Better Newsletter
8830 Glencoe Drive
Riverside, CA 92503
Request: Equipment Reviews
and Sources.

**Mountain People's
Warehouse**
P.O. Box 1027
Nevada City, CA 95959
(916) 273-9531
Carries about everything
including dairy products,
yogurts, kefirs, Evert-Fresh
Bags (see pp. 137-38). A
good resource for food co-
ops in Western states.
Services: California, Oregon,
Nevada, Idaho, Utah.

The Health Crest Company
295 Distribution Street
P.O. Box 1743
San Marcos, CA 92069
(619) 752-5230
UPS shipping nationwide.
COD and UPS COD orders
by phone accepted.

Evert-Fresh Bags
(see pp. 137-38)
for fresh produce.
For information, call:
(713) 529-4593
In CA: 1-800-795-8808

**Dr. Donsbach's Superoxy
Food Wash**
The Rockland Corp.
Tulsa, OK 74128
1-800-421-7310

**Nature Clean All Purpose
Lotion**
1-800-USA-1252

PART 7

❤

Nutrient Data
Meal Plans
Recipes
Notes
Recommended
Reading
Recipe Index
More Cooking and Home Ideas
from Sue and Emilie

❤

Nutrient Data Basics

The example below explains how the nutrient data for the recipes and menu suggestions (pp. 312-74) was determined.

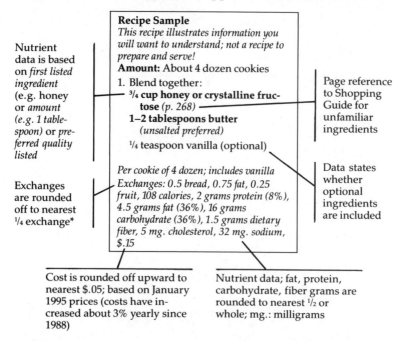

Nutrient data is based on *first listed ingredient* (e.g. honey or *amount* (e.g. 1 tablespoon) or *preferred quality listed*

Recipe Sample
This recipe illustrates information you will want to understand; not a recipe to prepare and serve!
Amount: About 4 dozen cookies
1. Blend together:
   ³/₄ cup honey or crystalline fructose *(p. 268)*
   1–2 tablespoons butter
   (unsalted preferred)
   ¹/₄ teaspoon vanilla (optional)

Per cookie of 4 dozen; includes vanilla Exchanges: 0.5 bread, 0.75 fat, 0.25 fruit, 108 calories, 2 grams protein (8%), 4.5 grams fat (36%), 16 grams carbohydrate (36%), 1.5 grams dietary fiber, 5 mg. cholesterol, 32 mg. sodium, $.15

Page reference to Shopping Guide for unfamiliar ingredients

Data states whether optional ingredients are included

Exchanges are rounded off to nearest ¹/₄ exchange*

Cost is rounded off upward to nearest $.05; based on January 1995 prices (costs have increased about 3% yearly since 1988)

Nutrient data; fat, protein, carbohydrate, fiber grams are rounded to nearest ¹/₂ or whole; mg.: milligrams

* Exchange values follow closely the values of Weight Watchers, American Diabetes Association, and other exchange programs. More information is available from *Eating Better Main Dishes* (see p. 384 for information).

Nutrient Data Sources

Nutrient data for this book has been compiled from *Sue's Nutridata © 1993* computer program based on the following sources (listed in order of first use where data available).

Available package labels

Total Nutrition Guide, Jean Carper, Bantam Books, 1989 (Complete and Up-to-date Based on USDA New Scientific Analysis of Vital Nutrients of More Than 2500 Foods).

Food Values of Portions Commonly Used, 14th Edition, Jean A.T. Pennington & Helen Nichols Church, Harper & Row, Publishers, 1985.

Nutrition Wizard, computer data program, Michael Jacobson, CSPI, 1986.

Nutrition Almanac, Revised Edition, Nutrition Search, Inc., John D. Kirschmann, Director, McGraw-Hill Book Company, 1979.

Laurel's Kitchen, Laurel Robertson, Carol Flinders & Bronwen Godfrey, Nilgiri Press, Berkeley, California, 1976.

Unlimited Meal Plan

Vegetarian Nondairy (Rice/Grain)	Ground Turkey	Vegetarian Dairy/Cheese	Fish	Vegetarian Bean	Vegetarian Nondairy (Potato) or Chicken	Vegetarian Dairy/Cheese
Brown Rice Pilaf (p. 313)	Favorite Tamalie Pie (p. 319)	Creamy Vegetable Chowder (p. 337)	Lemon Baked Fish (p. 346)	Lentil Rice Casserole (p. 315)	Baked Yam or Sweet Potato (p. 317) or Yams in Orange Sauce (p. 316)	Vegetable Lasagna (p. 334)
Marinated Tofu Stir-Fry (p. 340) or Stir-Fry Vegetables (p. 341) with Sweet 'n' Sour Sauce (p. 339) over Brown Rice (p. 312)	Turkey Burgers (p. 321) or Chili (p. 331) with Seasoned Ground Turkey (p. 320)	Eggplant Parmigiana (p. 325)	Almond Tuna Salad (p. 349) or Tuna Noodle Yummy (p. 345)	Black Bean Chowder (p. 335) or Emilie's 10-Bean Soup (p. 336)	Kid's Choice	Noodle Parmesan Supreme (p. 344)
Barley Casserole (p. 314) or Egg Real Fool! Sandwich (p. 353)	Emilie's Best Lasagna (p. 323) or Saucy Spaghetti with Seasoned Ground Turkey (p. 324)	5-Minute Blender Waffles (p. 355) or Golden Waffles/Pancakes (p. 354)	Dad's Choice	Chili (p. 331) or Chili Gourmet (p. 330) or Country Creole Peas 'n' Corn (p. 332)	Baked Parmesan Chicken (p. 350) or Cashew Chicken (p. 351)	Little Cottage Enchiladas (p. 343)
Dine Out	Sausage Strata (p. 322) or Ragout (p. 352)	Vegi Burrito Rollups (p. 326) with Tomato Soup (p. 327)	Lemon Baked Salmon (p. 348)	Split Pea Soup (p. 328) or Middle Eastern Lentil Soup (p. 329)	Ratatouille over Baked Potato (p. 333) or Golden Stuffed Potatoes (p. 317)	Sweet 'n' Sour Tofu Stir-Fry (p. 338) over Brown Rice (p. 312)

No-Meat Meal Plan (Lacto-Ovo-Vegetarian*)
(meats, fish, poultry excluded)

Vegetarian Dairy/Cheese	Vegetarian Nondairy (Grain)	Vegetarian Bean	Vegetarian Dairy/Cheese (Pasta)	Vegetarian Bean	Vegetarian Nondairy (Potato)	Vegetarian Dairy/Cheese
Vegi Burrito Rollups (p. 326) with Tomato Soup (p. 327)	Brown Rice Pilaf (p. 313)	Country Creole Peas 'n' Corn (p. 332) or Middle Eastern Lentil Soup (p. 329)	Noodle Parmesan Supreme (p. 344)	Black Bean Chowder (p. 335) or Emilie's 10-Bean Soup (p. 336)	Golden Stuffed Potatoes (p. 318)	Dine Out
Little Cottage Enchiladas (p. 343)	Barley Casserole (p. 314)	Split Pea Soup (p. 328)	Saucy Spaghetti (p. 324)	Savory Leftovers	Baked Yam or Sweet Potato (p. 317) or Yams in Orange Sauce (p. 316)	Creamy Vegetable Chowder (p. 337)
Eggplant Parmigiana (p. 325)	Stir-Fry Vegetables (p. 341) with Sweet 'n' Sour Sauce (p. 339) or Marinated Tofu Stir-Fry (p. 340)	Chili (p. 331) or Chili Gourmet (p. 330)	*Vegetable Lasagna (p. 334)	Lentil Rice Casserole (p. 315)	Ratatouille (p. 333) over Baked Potato	*5-Minute Blender Waffles (p. 355) or *Golden Waffles/Pancakes (p. 354)

* For a Lacto-Vegetarian Meal Plan (excluding eggs): These dishes represent complete menus. Some items on suggested menus, therefore, may need to be changed or an egg substitute used for a completely eggless menu. Three main dishes on this meal plan contain eggs. For a plan excluding eggs, there are several other eggless, meatless main dishes to substitute.

No-Dairy, No-Egg Meal Plan

Vegetarian Bean	Vegetarian Nondairy (Potato)	Chicken, Fish	Vegetarian Bean	Vegetarian Nondairy (Grain)	Ground Turkey	Vegetarian (Tofu, Pasta)
Lentil Rice Casserole (p. 315)	Golden Stuffed Potatoes (p. 318)	Lemon Baked Fish (p. 346)		Barley Casserole (p. 314)	Turkey Burgers (p. 321) or Ragout (p. 352)	Marinated Tofu Stir-Fry (p. 340)
Chili (p. 331) or Chili Gourmet (p. 330)	Baked Yam or Sweet Potato (p. 317) or Yams in Orange Sauce (p. 316)	Cashew Chicken (p. 351)	Emilie's 10-Bean Soup (p. 336) or Country Creole Peas 'n' Corn (p. 332)	Stir-Fry Vegetables (p. 341) with Sweet 'n' Sour Sauce (p. 339) over Brown Rice (p. 312)	Leftovers or Dine Out	Saucy Spaghetti (p. 324)
Middle Eastern Lentil Soup (p. 329)	Ratatouille (p. 333) over Baked Potato	Lemon Baked Salmon (p. 348)	Split Pea Soup (p. 328)	Brown Rice Pilaf (p. 313)	Favorite Tamalie Pie (p. 319)	Egg Real Fool! Sandwich (p. 353)

NOTE: These dishes represent complete menus. Some accompanying items on suggested menus, therefore, may need to be changed or a nondairy ingredient substituted for a complete nondairy menu.

BROWN RICE

Chewy and flavorful, about three times the dietary fiber of white rice and richer in calcium, phosphorus, potassium, and niacin. Of all the methods I have tried for cooking brown rice without a rice cooker, this method works best for me. To prepare in a rice cooker, use the same proportion of rice, water, and salt. The texture of long-grain brown rice is usually more pleasing to those used to eating white rice than short-grain or medium-grain brown rice. For a time-saver make extra rice to freeze in Ziploc freezer bags.

AMOUNT: 3 cups (4 to 6 servings)

1. Place in saucepan and bring to a boil:

   2¹/₂ cups water
   1 cup long-grain brown rice
   1 teaspoon salt *(RealSalt preferred, p. 269)* **or 2 teaspoons** *Sue's "Kitchen Magic"* *(see note below)*

2. Boil uncovered for 5 minutes.

3. Lower heat to very low, cover with a tight-fitting lid, and simmer 45-60 minutes, until tender and water is absorbed.

4. Do not uncover during cooking! Do not stir during cooking (may develop sticky rice).

1 serving (¹/₂ cup)

Exchanges: 1.5 bread
111 calories, 2.5 grams protein (8%), 0.5 grams fat (5%)
24 grams carbohydrate (87%), 1 gram dietary fiber
0 mg. cholesterol, 358 mg. sodium, $.05

Sue's "Kitchen Magic" Seasoning *is a special soy protein blend with alfalfa, corn, and wheat. It contains no MSG. It imparts a fantastic flavor to many recipes as an alternative to chicken broth. In fact, it tastes better! It is not sodium-free, but does reduce the need for salt and is lower in sodium than most commercial salted chicken broths and bouillon. One teaspoon contains 710 mg. sodium compared to 2132 mg. in a teaspoon of salt. It is an all-vegetable product. This seasoning is available by mail order from* **Eating Better Cookbooks** *(p. 383).*

BROWN RICE PILAF

*One of our company favorites from **Main Dishes**, we serve this often with **Baked Parmesan Chicken**. For a second meal I often add bits of leftover chicken and freeze it for a complete "dinner's ready" main dish. I also freeze it just as it is for a meatless menu. **Sue's "Kitchen Magic"** (p. 383) gives this dish its best flavor.*

AMOUNT: 6 servings

1. Combine together in saucepan, bring to a boil, and boil uncovered for 5 minutes:

    1¹/₂ cups uncooked long-grain brown rice
    ¹/₄ cup chopped, sliced, or slivered almonds
    3 cups water with 4 teaspoons *Sue's "Kitchen Magic"* (p. 383) **(or chicken broth)**
    2 teaspoons soy sauce (Kikkoman Lite preferred, p. 269)
    ¹/₈ teaspoon garlic powder

2. Cover with tight-fitting lid, reduce heat to low, and simmer 50-60 minutes or until all the water is absorbed. Do not remove lid during cooking and do not stir (may cause sticky rice).

3. While rice cooks, sauté for 1-2 minutes in 2 or 3 tablespoons water:

    2 green onions, chopped

4. Fold onions into cooked rice just before serving.

1 serving (about ³/₄ cup)

Exchanges: 2.5 bread, 0.5 fat
211 calories, 5 grams protein (10%), 4 grams fat (17%)
39 grams carbohydrate (73%), 2 grams dietary fiber
0 mg. cholesterol, 543 mg. sodium, $.20

VARIATIONS

♥ Replace ¹/₄ cup of the rice with **¹/₄ cup wild rice or wheat kernels.**

♥ For gourmet touch, brown the rice and almonds over medium heat, stirring frequently, in ¹/₄ **cup melted butter.**

MENU SUGGESTION (445 calories, 19% fat, $1.05):
Brown Rice Pilaf—1 serving
Broccoli (p. 362)—1 cup
Mexi-Salad—2¹/₂-3 cups (lettuce, romaine, kidney beans, cheddar cheese, tomato) with *Sweet Lite Dressing* (p. 373)—2 tablespoons

---

BARLEY CASSEROLE

A hearty dish from **Casseroles** *that is truly vegetarian when water and* **Sue's** *"Kitchen Magic," p. 383, are used in place of broth. Why not double the recipe and freeze an extra casserole for a later meal? Note the very low fat content!*

AMOUNT: 6 servings
Bake: 350° for 1¹/₂–2 hours, covered

1. Brown over medium heat, stirring frequently for about 10 minutes:

   ³/₄ cup pearl barley, uncooked

2. Lightly sauté in 2 or 3 tablespoons water:

   ¹/₂ onion, chopped
   1 rib celery, chopped
   1 small green pepper, chopped

3. Bring to a boil in a saucepan:

   2 cups water with 1¹/₂ teaspoons *Sue's "Kitchen Magic"* (p. 383)
      (or chicken or beef broth)
   2 teaspoons soy sauce (Kikkoman Lite preferred, p. 269)

4. Pour hot broth into 9″ x 13″ pan or casserole dish; mix in:

   browned barley
   sautéed vegetables
   1 cup fresh mushrooms, sliced
   small (8³/₄ oz.) can garbanzo beans, drained, rinsed
   ¹/₂ of 8-oz. can water chestnuts, sliced and drained

5. Cover and bake at 350° for 1¹/₂–2 hours until barley is tender and liquid is absorbed.

1 serving

Exchanges: 1.75 bread, 1 vegetable
152 calories, 5.5 grams protein (13%), 1 gram fat (6%)
33 grams carbohydrate (81%), 2.5 grams dietary fiber
0 mg. cholesterol, 349 mg. sodium, $.35

MENU SUGGESTION (609 calories, 11% fat, $1.70)
Barley Casserole—1 serving
Broccoli-Carrot Medley with Lemon Butter (p. 363)—1 serving
Tossed salad—2 cups (leafy lettuce, red cabbage, celery, carrot, tomato, radishes) with *Sweet Orange Dressing* (p. 373)
Whole-grain rolls—2 with 100% fruit jam—2 tablespoons

LENTIL RICE CASSEROLE

*Takes five minutes to assemble. One of our **Main Dishes** recipes most often requested! Meatless and low cost. Lentils and brown rice mutually increase the protein value of the other. **Sue's "Kitchen Magic,"** p. 383, gives this dish its best flavor! Our favorite way to serve it is "hidden" in burritos. Freezes well. (Demonstrated on "**Eating Better with Sue**" video, p. 383)*

AMOUNT: about 3 cups (4 to 6 servings)
Bake: 300° for 2–2¹/₂ hours, covered

1. Blend together in a casserole dish:

   ³/₄ **cup uncooked lentils, green or red**
   ¹/₂ **cup uncooked long-grain brown rice**
   ¹/₄ **cup instant minced onion (or 1 small chopped onion)**
   3 cups water with 1 tablespoon *Sue's "Kitchen Magic"* (p. 383)
     (or chicken broth)
   ¹/₂ **teaspoon basil leaves**
   ¹/₄ **teaspoon oregano leaves**
   ¹/₄ **teaspoon thyme leaves**
   ¹/₄ **teaspoon garlic powder**

2. Cover and bake for 2–2¹/₂ hours at 300°.

3. During last 20 minutes of baking top with:

   ¹/₂ **cup grated cheddar cheese** (optional)

4. Just before serving, stir to blend in the melted cheese. If desired garnish with:

   a handful of minced fresh parsley

¹/₂ cup without cheese

Exchanges: 0.25 meat, 1.75 bread, 0.5 vegetable
153 calories, 7.5 grams protein (20%), 0.5 gram fat (4%)
29 grams carbohydrate (76%), 4 grams dietary fiber
0 mg. cholesterol, 367 mg. sodium, $.20

¹/₂ cup with cheese

Exchanges: 0.5 meat, 1.75 bread, 0.5 fat, 0.5 vegetable
191 calories, 10 grams protein (23%), 4 grams fat (18%)
29 grams carbohydrate (61%), 4 grams dietary fiber
10 mg. cholesterol, 382 mg. sodium, $.30

MENU SUGGESTION (793 calories, 22% fat, $1.40)
Lentil rice burritos—2 (2 whole-wheat tortillas, 1 cup leafy lettuce, 1 chopped tomato, salsa, 2 tablespoons light sour cream, 1 cup Lentil Rice Casserole with cheese)
Carrot and celery sticks—4 each

YAMS IN ORANGE SAUCE

A favorite Thanksgiving or Christmas dish, but good anytime! The sweet sauce minimizes the need for excessive butter.

AMOUNT: 6 to 8 servings
Bake: 375° for 45 minutes; then 350° for 30 minutes, covered

1. Set on oven rack and bake at 375° about 45 minutes until almost tender (see baking tip, p. 288):

   6 medium yams or sweet potatoes

2. Peel and slice yams into lightly buttered casserole dish.

3. Blend together and pour over top of yams:

   1 cup orange juice
   ¼ cup honey or crystalline fructose (p. 268)
   2 tablespoons melted butter (unsalted preferred)
   2 tablespoons arrowroot powder (p. 268) **or cornstarch**

4. Cover and bake at 350° for 30 minutes.

1 serving of 6
Exchanges: 2.75 bread, 0.75 fat, 0.25 fruit
258 calories, 3 grams protein (5%), 4 grams fat (14%)
54 grams carbohydrate (81%), 3 grams dietary fiber
10 mg. cholesterol, 18 mg. sodium, $.40

MENU SUGGESTION (465 calories, 22% fat, $.75)
Yams in Orange Sauce—1 serving of 6
Frozen green peas—½ cup
Waldorf salad (½ apple, 1 rib celery, 1 tablespoon each raisins, walnuts) with *Sweet Lite Dressing* (p. 373)—1 tablespoon
Sourdough bread—1 slice with *Butter Spread* (p. 371)—1½ teaspoons

BAKED YAM OR SWEET POTATO

A potato can be a filling main dish. Yams sold in the United States are a variety of sweet potato. A true yam is very low in nutrients while 1 cup mashed sweet potato contains about 16,000 IU's provitamin A (see p. 139), 49 mg. vitamin C, 56 mg. calcium, and 696 mg. potassium. Eat the skins just like Irish and new potato skins for an unusual treat and added fiber.

AMOUNT: as desired
Bake: 400° for 1 hour

Scrub and cut small slice off ends to prevent bursting of skins; set on oven rack and bake at 400° about 1 hour or until done:

1 baking potato (about 8 oz.) per person

Baking Tip: Set a piece of foil over bottom of oven when baking yams or sweet potatoes to catch possible spills from bursting skins.

1 serving (8-oz. potato)

Exchanges: 3.25 bread
237 calories, 4 grams protein (6%), less than 0.5 gram fat (1%)
55 grams carbohydrate (93%), 4 grams dietary fiber
0 mg. cholesterol, 23 mg. sodium, $.35

1 serving (8-oz. potato) with 1 tablespoon **Butter Spread***, p. 371*

Exchanges: 3.25 bread, 2.5 fat
347 calories, 4 grams protein (4%), 13 grams fat (33%)
55 grams carbohydrate (63%), 4 grams dietary fiber
16 mg. cholesterol, 81 mg. sodium, $.40

MENU SUGGESTION (776 calories, 30% fat, $1.40)
Baked Yam or Sweet Potato—1 serving
   with *Butter Spread* (p. 371)—1 tablespoon
Snappy Bean Salad (p. 361)—1 serving
Fresh pineapple wedge—about 2½ oz.
Whole-grain rolls—1½ with 100% fruit jam—1 tablespoon

GOLDEN STUFFED POTATOES

A tasty alternative to butter-laden potatoes! These make a big hit when served to company. Serve with no extra butter at the table. Serve as main dish for vegetarian meal or with any meat dish. Each stuffed half provides 32% of the RDA of vitamin A and 39% of vitamin C.

AMOUNT: 3–4 servings (1½-2 halves each)
Bake: 400° for 1 hour; 350° for 10-15 minutes, covered

1. Wash, set on oven rack, and bake at 400° until done, about 1 hour:

   3 baking-size (8 oz.) potatoes

2. Meanwhile, cut into 3" chunks:

   about 1 lb. banana squash or yellow squash, seeds removed, to make 1¼ cups mashed cooked squash

3. Place squash skin-side-down in vegetable steamer over boiling water, cover, and steam until very tender, about 20-30 minutes.

4. When squash is still very warm but cool enough to handle, scoop it from skin with a spoon into electric mixer bowl (if you have one—otherwise into regular mixing bowl).

5. While baked potatoes are still hot but cool enough to handle, cut in half lengthwise and scoop potato with spoon into bowl with the squash.

6. Add:

   1 tablespoon soft butter *(unsalted preferred)*
   1 teaspoon salt *(RealSalt preferred, p. 269)*
   ³/₈-½ teaspoon ground cumin seed, to taste *(p. 269)*

7. Blend until smooth with electric beaters or potato masher. Pile potato-squash mixture into potato shells. Garnish with paprika. Place in covered pan or casserole and return to oven to heat through.

½ stuffed potato

Exchanges: 1.5 bread, 0.5 fat, 0.5 vegetable
156 calories, 3 grams protein (7%), 2.5 grams fat (14%)
32 grams carbohydrate (79%), 5 grams dietary fiber
5 mg. cholesterol, 364 mg. sodium, $.45

MENU SUGGESTION (690 calories, 18% fat, $1.20)
Golden Stuffed Potatoes—2 halves
Amandine green beans (½ cup beans, 1 tablespoon almonds, ³/₄ teaspoon butter)
Fruit coleslaw (cabbage, carrot, apple, pineapple, raisins) with *Sweet Lite Dressing (p. 373)*—1 tablespoon

---

FAVORITE TAMALIE PIE

One of our best-loved freezer meals from **Casseroles!**

AMOUNT: 6 servings
Bake: 350° for 50-60 minutes, uncovered

1. Season and brown *(p. 320)*:
   1 lb. ground turkey *(90% fat free)*

2. When turkey is about half browned, add and sauté until turkey is cooked:
   1 small green pepper, chopped
   1 small onion, chopped
   1 clove garlic, minced

3. Lower heat and blend in:
   2—8-oz. cans (2 cups) tomato sauce
   2 cups corn, frozen or fresh
   2.25-oz. can sliced ripe olives, drained (optional)
   1½ teaspoons chili powder
   ½ teaspoon salt *(RealSalt preferred, p. 269)*

4. Pour hot mixture into 9″ square baking pan or 2-quart casserole dish.

5. *For topping* bring to boil in saucepan:
   1 cup water
   ½ teaspoon salt *(RealSalt preferred, p. 269)*
   1 tablespoon butter *(unsalted preferred)*

6. In separate bowl blend cornmeal into a second cup of water:
   1 cup cold water
   1 cup stoneground cornmeal *(p. 267)*

7. Gradually stir cold water-cornmeal mixture into boiling water, stirring to thicken, about 2 minutes. Spread cooked cornmeal mixture evenly to edges over top of casserole.

8. Bake uncovered for 50-60 minutes at 350° or until crust is done (lightly crisp and golden brown).

1 serving with optional olives

Exchanges: 2.5 meat, 1.75 bread, 0.75 fat, 1.75 vegetable
340 calories, 26 grams protein (29%), 12 grams fat (30%)
37 grams carbohydrate (41%), 8 grams dietary fiber
53 mg. cholesterol, 1051 mg. sodium, $.90

MENU SUGGESTION (660 calories, 18% fat, $1.90):
Favorite Tamalie Pie—1 serving
Orange slices—3, pineapple slices—2, on leaf lettuce with *Sweet Lite Dressing (p. 373)*—2 tablespoons
Cooked Broccoli *(p. 362)*—1 cup, or other green vegetable
Whole-grain roll—1 with 100% fruit jam—1 tablespoon

SEASONED GROUND TURKEY

*Ground turkey is lower in fat, cholesterol, and calories than ground beef. You can learn more about different fat levels of ground turkey as compared to different types of ground beef from **Main Dishes**. We use it entirely in place of ground beef. The seasoning is so easy and really improves the flavor! Demonstrated on the **"Eating Better with Sue"** video (see p. 383). Cooked seasoned ground turkey freezes well for use in any casserole.*

AMOUNT: 1 lb.

1. Stir together thoroughly with a fork and brown in frying pan:

   1 lb. ground turkey *(90% fat free)*
   1 tablespoon soy sauce *(Kikkoman Lite preferred, p. 269)*
   2 tablespoons tomato sauce or catsup *(no salt added, p. 268)*
   1/8 teaspoon nutmeg
   1/8 teaspoon thyme leaves
   1/8 teaspoon garlic powder
   1/8 teaspoon sage

1 lb. seasoned (90% fat free*)

Exchanges: 14.5 meat, 0.5 vegetable
894 calories, 126 grams protein (55%), 44 grams fat (43%)
5 grams carbohydrate (2%), 289 mg. cholesterol, 642 mg. sodium, $2.40

> * *Labeling tip:* Food companies choose labeling terms to cast their products in the best possible light. For example "90% fat free" means the product contains 10% fat by weight. By calories, however, it contains 45% fat (45% of the calories come from fat). Some confusing labeling practices will be better controlled by the new labeling law (see p. 293).

GROUND TURKEY SEASONING MIX

Keep a blend of spices and herbs for seasoning ground turkey on hand for quick use. Label the container: "Use 1/2 teaspoon per 1 lb. + 2 tablespoons catsup + 1 tablespoon soy sauce."

AMOUNT: seasons 48 lbs. ground turkey

1. Blend together thoroughly and store in tightly covered labeled container in kitchen cupboard:

   2 tablespoons nutmeg
   2 tablespoons thyme leaves
   2 tablespoons garlic powder
   2 tablespoons sage

2. Use 1/2 **teaspoon seasoning mix per lb.**

TURKEY BURGER PATTIES

Seasoned Ground Turkey shaped into patties! Add the bran for extra nutrition and to help hold patties more firmly together. To freeze, place pieces of waxed paper between patties, wrap in saran, then snuggle in foil.

AMOUNT: 4 patties

1. Mix together thoroughly with a fork:
    1 lb. *Seasoned Ground Turkey* (p. 320)
    ½-¾ cup oat bran (optional)
2. Shape 4 burger patties.
3. Bake in oven at 350° for 10-15 minutes in a shallow pan. These may also be fried, but are not as moist this way. No fat is needed to cook turkey burger in any pan.

Barbecue tip: To barbecue, set patties in foil cupped around the edges; otherwise meat will fall through grill.

1 patty (includes oat bran)
Exchanges: 3.75 meat, 0.5 bread
257 calories, 33.5 grams protein (50%), 11.5 grams fat (39%)
8 grams carbohydrate (11%), 3 grams dietary fiber
72 mg. cholesterol, 162 mg. sodium, $.65

TURKEY BURGERS

Turkey is native to America, so the true "all-American" burger is a turkey burger!

AMOUNT: 1 turkey burger

Assemble, as desired:
    1 whole-grain hamburger bun (p. 267)
    1 *Turkey Burger Patty* (above)
    2 tablespoons *Thousand Island Dressing* (p. 372)
    1 thick slice of large tomato
    1 slice onion
    ¼ cup alfalfa sprouts
    leafy green lettuce

1 burger
Exchanges: 3.75 meat, 4.25 bread, 2 fat, 1 vegetable
683 calories, 46 grams protein (26%), 23.5 grams fat (30%)
76 grams carbohydrate (43%), 12.5 grams dietary fiber
93 mg. cholesterol, 617 mg. sodium, $1.10

> **MENU SUGGESTION** (789 calories, 26% fat, $1.35):
> *Turkey Burger*—1
> Carrot sticks—4, celery sticks—4, cucumber slices—6
> Apple—1

SAUSAGE STRATA

A freezer dish from **Casseroles** *with sausage flavor (the "secret" is the nutmeg). Compare the high fat percentage of calories of this recipe (51%) with the menu suggestion below (29%). This illustrates how the actual percentage of fat consumed in a meal can be altered by the choice of other menu items.*

AMOUNT: 6 servings
Bake: 350° for 30 minutes, covered

1. Lightly sauté zucchini in oil; remove and set aside:
   - **2 tablespoons olive oil**
   - **4 generous cups unpeeled zucchini slices**

2. Mix together and brown in same pan:
   - **1 lb. ground turkey** (90% fat free)
   - **1 small onion, chopped**
   - **1 teaspoon salt** (RealSalt preferred, p. 269)
   - **1/2 teaspoon nutmeg**
   - **1/2 teaspoon sage**
   - **1/2 teaspoon thyme leaves**
   - **1/16-1/8 teaspoon cayenne pepper, to taste**

3. For *cheese sauce*, whisk cornstarch into cold milk and whisk into hot milk. Whisk constantly until thickened, about 2 minutes (do not boil). Blend in cheese:
   - **1/4 cup cold low-fat milk**
   - **2 tablespoons cornstarch**
   - **1 1/4 cups hot low-fat milk**
   - **1 cup grated cheddar cheese**

4. Combine with turkey mixture:
   - **3 eggs, beaten with a fork**
   - **1 cup whole-wheat bread crumbs (1 slice in blender)**
   - **1/8 teaspoon garlic powder**

5. Layer cheese sauce, zucchini slices, and turkey mixture in baking dish in 2 layers. Start and end with cheese sauce. Garnish with **parsley**. Cover and bake at 350° for 30 minutes.

1 Serving

Exchanges: 3.5 meat, 0.5 milk, 0.5 bread, 2 fat, 1 vegetable
396 calories, 34 grams protein (33%), 23 grams fat (51%), 16 grams carbohydrate (16%), 1.5 grams dietary fiber 181 mg. cholesterol, 546 mg. sodium, $.95

MENU SUGGESTION (776 calories, 29% fat, $1.75):
Sausage Strata—1 serving; frozen peas—1/2 cup
Carrot combo salad (grated carrot, raisins, apple, pineapple, celery) with *Sweet Lite Dressing* (p. 373)—1 tablespoon
Whole-grain rolls—1 1/2 with 100% fruit jam—1 tablespoon

EMILIE'S BEST LASAGNA

*Emilie's best lasagna and no precooking noodles! She serves this **Holiday Menus** recipe during the Christmas season to a crowd of young adults. It is always a party hit! Serve with a big salad, olive oil dressing, and dessert.*

AMOUNT: 6 to 8 servings (9" x 13" pan)
Bake: 350° for 1 hour, uncovered

1. Brown in frying pan (no oil, but spray lightly with olive oil nonstick spray, if desired):
   2 cloves garlic, minced
   1 lb. ground turkey seasoned according to recipe for *Sausage Strata*, **p. 322, step #2—omit the onion or use 1 lb. Italian turkey sausage** *(from supermarket)*

2. Stir in and simmer while preparing remaining ingredients:
   1 tablespoon basil leaves *(if possible, use fresh)*
   28-oz. or 29-oz. can tomato puree or sauce
   6-oz. can tomato paste

3. Meanwhile, mix together:
   2 eggs, beaten
   3 cups skim milk ricotta cheese
   ½ cup grated Parmesan cheese
   2 tablespoons dried parsley flakes or ¼ cup fresh minced
   1 teaspoon salt *(RealSalt preferred, p. 269)*
   ½ teaspoon pepper

4. Slice thinly:
   1 lb. mozzarella cheese

5. Spread ¼ cup sauce evenly over bottom of 9" x 13" baking pan.

6. Make 3 layers of ingredients in order given. Bake uncovered at 350° for 1 hour until noodles are tender.
   8 oz. uncooked whole-grain lasagna noodles *(p. 267)*
   ricotta cheese mixture
   tomato sauce
   mozzarella cheese

1 serving of 8

Exchanges: 5.75 meat, 0.5 milk, 1.25 bread, 0.25 fat, 1.5 vegetable
526 calories, 50 grams protein (36%), 22.5 grams fat (37%)
37 grams carbohydrate (27%), 4.5 grams dietary fiber
125 mg. cholesterol, 1673 mg. sodium, $1.70

MENU SUGGESTION (787 calories, 30% fat, $2.80)
Emilie's Best Lasagna—1 serving of 8
Green salad—2 cups (lettuce greens, celery, bell pepper, zucchini, green onion, cherry tomatoes) with *Emilie's Olive Oil Dressing* *(p. 372)*—½ tablespoon
Frozen Vanilla Yogurt (p. 370)—¾ cup with *Pineapple Topping (p. 370)*—¼ cup

SAUCY SPAGHETTI

Why not try it meatless? Experiment with different kinds of whole-grain pasta besides whole wheat from the health-food store such as corn, quinoa, spelt, or Kamut. Kamut is especially light and highest of the grains in protein and minerals. If you can find it, you will undoubtedly like it best!

AMOUNT: 6 servings

1. Sauté in a little olive oil, or simmer in a little water 5-10 minutes:

   1 green pepper, chopped
   1 onion, chopped
   2 cloves garlic, minced
   1 cup fresh mushrooms, sliced

2. Add to drained vegetables and simmer 30 minutes:

   28-oz. can tomato pieces or 2 12-oz. cans tomato sauce
   6-oz. can tomato paste
   1 teaspoon Italian seasoning, to taste

3. Meanwhile bring water to a boil, add spaghetti, and cook just until tender, according to time given on package directions:

   4 quarts water
   1 teaspoon olive oil
   ¹/₄ teaspoon salt *(RealSalt preferred, p. 269)*
   8-oz. package whole-grain spaghetti *(p. 267)*

4. Top sauce over spaghetti with **Parmesan cheese**, if desired.

1 serving (oil for step 1 and Parmesan cheese not included)

Exchanges: 1.5 bread, 0.25 fat, 3 vegetable
186 calories, 7 grams protein (15%), 2.5 grams fat (11%)
37 grams carbohydrate (74%), 6 grams dietary fiber
0 mg. cholesterol, 566 mg. sodium, $.70

VARIATIONS

♥ Add **1 lb.** browned *Seasoned Ground Turkey* (p. 320)
♥ Add **2 cups cooked kidney beans or lentils.**

1 serving with Seasoned Ground Turkey (90% fat free)

Exchanges: 2.5 meat, 1.5 bread, 0.25 fat, 3 vegetable
335 calories, 28 grams protein (32%), 10 grams fat (25%)
37 grams carbohydrate (42%), 6 grams dietary fiber

MENU SUGGESTION: (569 calories, 30% fat, $1.70):
Saucy Spaghetti (meatless)—1 serving with Parmesan cheese—
  2 tablespoons
Green beans—³/₄ cup
Tossed salad—2 cups (leafy lettuce, red cabbage, celery, carrot,
  tomato, radishes) with *Sweet Orange Dressing* (p. 373)
Sourdough bread—2 with *Butter Spread* (p. 371)—1 tablespoon

EGGPLANT PARMIGIANA

We enjoy the Gourmet Variation of this recipe with a little firmer eggplant, but many enjoy the very soft eggplant version as well, which is quicker to prepare and lower in fat. The Gourmet Variation menu below is 27% fat.

AMOUNT: 6 servings
Bake: 350° for 20 minutes, uncovered

1. Lightly salt eggplant slices on both sides, let stand 30 minutes, and rinse thoroughly:

   1 medium eggplant, ¹/₄"-³/₈" slices, peeled or unpeeled

2. Steam eggplant slices 5-10 minutes until fork tender, but not enough to fall apart (unpeeled slices take a bit longer).

3. Coat eggplant slices in cornmeal:

   1 cup stoneground cornmeal *(p. 267)*

4. In lightly greased baking pan layer eggplant with remaining ingredients in 2 or 3 layers, beginning with eggplant, then sauce, cheeses, basil:

   2 cups spaghetti or tomato sauce
   1¹/₂ cups mozzarella cheese, grated
   ¹/₄ cup Parmesan cheese
   2 teaspoons basil leaves

5. Bake uncovered about 20 minutes at 350° or until cheese melts and sauce is heated through.

1 serving

Exchanges: 1.75 meat, 1 bread, 1.75 vegetable
226 calories, 14 grams protein (24%), 8 grams fat (30%)
27 grams carbohydrate (56%), 5 grams dietary fiber
20 mg. cholesterol, 699 mg. sodium, $.70

GOURMET VARIATION: Eggplant will be a little firmer. Do not steam eggplant. Dip slices into **2 eggs, slightly beaten**, then cornmeal. Brown slices in **olive oil, as needed**. Drain well on paper towels.

1 serving (with ¹/₄ cup oil, 2 eggs):

Exchanges: 2.25 meat, 1 bread, 2 fat, 1.75 vegetable
332 calories, 16 grams protein (1%), 19 grams fat (49%)
28 grams carbohydrate (32%), 5 grams dietary fiber
91 mg. cholesterol, 722 mg. sodium, $.80

MENU SUGGESTION (628 calories, 17% fat, $1.85):
Eggplant Parmigiana—1 serving
Orange tossed salad—2 cups (leafy lettuce, orange chunks, chopped celery) with *Sweet Lite Dressing* *(p. 373)*—1 tablespoon
Green beans—¹/₂ cup
Whole-grain rolls—2, or bread with 100% fruit jam—2 tablespoons

---

VEGI BURRITO ROLLUPS

Very tasty! Use this basic idea with a variety of vegetables (avocado, jicama, cauliflowerets, etc.). Leftover burritos may be wrapped in plastic wrap to eat cold the next day.

AMOUNT: 8 burritos
Bake: 300° for 10 minutes, covered lightly

1. Mix together:

>   **1 sliced onion, sautéed in a little water, drained**
>   **2 cups cooked broccoli, very small pieces** *(p. 362)*
>   **¼ cup barbecue sauce** *(p. 268)*
>   **2 medium carrots (³/₄-1 cup), grated fine**
>   **½ cup red cabbage, chopped or shredded fine**
>   **¼ cup fresh parsley, chopped fine**
>   **1 dill pickle, chopped fine**
>   **½ teaspoon Spike Seasoning** *(p. 269)*

2. Blend together in a separate bowl:

>   **½ cup nonfat plain yogurt**
>   **½ cup light sour cream**

3. Lay tortillas or chapatis out on waxed paper one at a time and fill each with the remaining ingredients in order given:

>   **8 whole-grain tortillas** *(p. 267)* **or chapatis**
>   **2 tablespoons yogurt and sour cream mixture** (spread out in center of tortilla with back of a spoon)
>   **about ½ cup vegetable mixture** (spread a bit with spoon)
>   **about ½ cup alfalfa sprouts** (if desired, reserve for garnish)

4. Roll up tortillas or fold over and secure each with a toothpick. Set in 9" x 13" bake pan, cover lightly with foil and heat about 10 minutes at 300°.

5. Garnish on serving plates, as desired with:

>   **shredded lettuce**
>   **tomato and/or avocado wedges or chunks**
>   **mound of alfalfa sprouts**

1 rollup with whole-wheat tortilla (garnishes not included)

Exchanges: 0.25 milk, 2.25 bread, 0.25 fat, 1.75 vegetable
224 calories, 9.5 grams protein (17%), 6 grams fat (23%)
34.5 grams carbohydrate (60%), 6 grams dietary fiber
5 mg. cholesterol, 109 mg. sodium, $.50

MENU SUGGESTION (681 calories, 26% fat, $1.75):
Vegi Burrito Rollups—2, with 1 cup lettuce, ¼ avocado
Tomato Soup, Lite Variation *(p. 327)*—2 cups
Fresh pineapple wedges—2 (about 5 oz.)

TOMATO SOUP

My favorite quick soup from **Soups & Muffins** *when I don't feel like cooking. A five-minute assembly operation, and so-o-o good! Freezes well.*

AMOUNT: about 15 cups (7 to 10 servings)

1. Blend together in soup pot and heat until very hot:

   10 cups water
   12-oz. can (1¹/₂ cups) tomato paste
   28-oz. can (3¹/₂ cups) tomato pieces
   ¹/₂ cup minced fresh parsley
   3 tablespoons honey
   2 teaspoons dill weed

2. Whisk milk and flour together until smooth; whisk into soup; cook and stir until thickened:

   1 cup low-fat or nonfat milk
   ³/₄ cup whole-wheat or whole-wheat pastry flour *(preferred, p. 267)* **or ¹/₂ cup unbleached white flour**

3. Season with:

   2 teaspoons salt, to taste *(RealSalt preferred, p. 269)*
   ¹/₄ cup (¹/₂ stick) unsalted butter (optional for added flavor)

1 cup (butter included)

Exchanges: 0.25 bread, 0.5 fat, 1.25 vegetable
102 calories, 3 grams protein (11%), 4 grams fat (32%)
16 grams carbohydrate (57%), 2 grams dietary fiber
10 mg. cholesterol, 587 mg. sodium, $.20

1 cup (excludes butter)

Exchanges: 0.25 bread, 1.25 vegetable
75 calories, 3 grams protein (14%), 1 gram fat (9%)
16 grams carbohydrate (77%), 2 grams dietary fiber
1 mg. cholesterol, 586 mg. sodium, $.20

LITE SOUP VARIATION
Omit milk and flour (step 2) and omit butter.

1 cup Lite Soup (excludes milk, flour, butter)

Exchanges: 1.5 vegetable
46 calories, 1.5 grams protein (13%), 0.5 gram fat (7%)
10.5 grams carbohydrate (80%), 1 gram dietary fiber
0 mg. cholesterol, 620 mg. sodium, $.20

MENU SUGGESTION (see Menu Suggestion, p. 326)

SPLIT PEA SOUP

A family favorite, familiar to everyone. Surprisingly tasty without ham bone. Freezes well. To make in Crockpot, combine all ingredients in pot except the salt and cook overnight on low or about 5-6 hours on high. Crockpot soup is not as rich and thick, but makes more because there is less evaporation of the water. I do it both ways, and we like it both ways.

AMOUNT: 4 to 6 servings

1. Bring peas and water to a boil; boil 3 minutes; reduce heat to a very gentle boil until peas are tender, 45-60 minutes (add more water, if needed):

   8 cups water
   2 cups split peas

2. Add and continue very gentle boil until vegetables are tender, about 15-20 minutes (add more water, if needed):

   1 medium onion, chopped
   3 medium carrots, diced or sliced
   3 ribs celery, chopped, or bunch of chopped celery leaves
   1 bay leaf
   1¼ teaspoons salt, to taste (RealSalt preferred, p. 269)

3. Remove bay leaf.

4. Puree part or all of soup in blender, as desired. Blending helps to thicken soup and increase flavor.

5. Garnish as desired with:

   grated cheddar, Jack, or Parmesan cheese
   Spike Seasoning (p. 269)
   Soup 'n' Salad Croutons (p. 361)

---

1 serving of 4 (garnishes not included)

Exchanges: 1 meat, 4.25 bread, 2 vegetable
394 calories, 26 grams protein (25%), 2 grams fat (4%)
74 grams carbohydrate (71%), 8.5 grams dietary fiber
0 mg. cholesterol, 768 mg. sodium, $.30

MENU SUGGESTION (747 calories, 9% fat, $1.20):
Split Pea Soup—1 serving of 4
Orange tossed salad—2 cups (leafy lettuce, orange chunks, chopped celery, banana slices) with *Sweet Lite Dressing* (p. 373)—1 tablespoon
Whole-Wheat Popovers (p. 358)—2 with 100% fruit jam—2 tablespoons

MIDDLE EASTERN LENTIL SOUP

Since I have a large Crockpot, I double this recipe. Mix everything together except the parsley and cheese, and cook on low overnight (8-10 hours). Lentils are tender by morning. This soup freezes well, as do most bean soups. I prefer to use Bragg Liquid Aminos (p. 268) in this soup. It is lower in sodium and milder in flavor than soy sauce.

AMOUNT: 4 to 6 servings (9 cups if made in Crockpot)

1. Bring to a boil for 3 minutes; reduce heat and simmer at a very gentle boil until lentils are tender, about 30-60 minutes:

   1½ cups lentils, dry
   7 cups water
   1 medium onion, chopped
   1 large or 2 medium ribs celery
   1 large or 2 medium carrots, sliced or diced
   1 clove garlic, minced

2. Puree half the soup (or more) in blender; pour back into soup pot and add:

   6 tablespoons Bragg Liquid Aminos (p. 268) **or 3 tablespoons soy sauce, to taste** (Kikkoman Lite preferred, p. 269)
   juice of 1 lemon (or about 4 teaspoons)
   1 teaspoon ground cumin seed (p. 269)
   1 tablespoon butter (unsalted preferred)

3. Simmer 15 minutes longer. Add 5-10 minutes before serving:

   ½ cup minced fresh parsley (optional)

4. Top each serving, if desired, with:

   ¼ cup grated cheddar or Jack cheese (optional)

1 serving of 4 (cheese garnish not included)

Exchanges: 1.25 meat, 2.75 bread, 0.5 fat, 1.75 vegetable
329 calories, 19 grams protein (25%), 4 grams fat (11%)
50 grams carbohydrate (64%), 12 grams dietary fiber
8 mg. cholesterol, 69 mg. sodium, $.55

MENU SUGGESTION (870 calories, 11% fat, $1.75):
Middle Eastern Lentil Soup—1 serving of 4
Pineapple Cornbread (p. 359)—2 pieces with honey—2 tablespoons
Vegetable munchies (zucchini sticks—4, cherry tomatoes—3, jicama sticks—4, green pepper strips—2, radish roses—2) with *Patty's Curry Dip* (p. 371)—2 tablespoons

---

CHILI GOURMET

A delightfully different chili with frozen tofu from **Casseroles**. *Even if you freeze the completed chili, do freeze the tofu before preparing the dish to get the best result of the texture change.*

AMOUNT: 6 to 8 servings (about 10 cups)

1. To prepare tofu, drain block, cover with fresh water, and freeze overnight. Thaw under running hot water, gradually pressing out the moisture and crumbling it as it thaws; set aside:

   About 14-oz. regular or firm block tofu (p. 269)

2. Sauté vegetables in oil (or a little water and drain); add tofu and remaining ingredients:

   2 tablespoons olive oil (optional)
   1 large green pepper, chopped
   2 cups fresh sliced mushrooms
   2 cloves minced garlic or ¹/₄ teaspoon garlic powder
   15.25-oz. can kidney beans, drained (*no salt added preferred*)
   27-oz. can kidney beans, drained (*no salt added preferred*)
   1¹/₂ cups water (or bean juice, if you prefer)
   2 14.5-oz cans (4 cups) tomato pieces or 2 15-oz. cans tomato sauce
   1 tablespoon chili powder
   1¹/₂ teaspoons ground cumin seed (p. 269)
   1 teaspoon salt, to taste (*RealSalt preferred, p. 269*)

3. Add water, if needed, to just cover ingredients. Bring to a boil, reduce to simmer, and cook briefly, about 10 minutes.

1 serving of 6 (includes olive oil):
Exchanges: 1 meat, 2 bread, 0.75 fat, 2.25 vegetable
305 calories, 15 grams protein (20%), 7.5 grams fat (22%)
44 grams carbohydrate (58%), 9.5 grams dietary fiber
0 mg. cholesterol, 396 mg. sodium, $1.15

VARIATION:
Replace canned beans with **2 cups dry kidney beans**. Cover with **8 cups water** in Crockpot and cook on low overnight or until tender; drain, reserving liquid to replace water in steps 2 and 3.

MENU SUGGESTION (856 calories, 12% fat, $1.85):
Chili Gourmet—1 serving (about 1²/₃ cups)
Pineapple Cornbread (p. 359)—2 pieces with honey—2 tablespoons
Carrot sticks—4, celery sticks—4
Apple—1 medium

CHILI

Chili without meat is really quite good! This dish from **Main Dishes** *freezes well. Canned tomato products and beans are typically very high in sodium. Consider unsalted or lower sodium products in recipes such as this. Salt to taste. The final result will probably be lower in sodium.*

AMOUNT: about 6 cups (3 to 4 servings)

1. Combine in saucepan:

> **15.25-oz. can kidney beans, drained** *(no salt added preferred)*
> **27-oz. can kidney beans, drained** *(no salt added preferred)*
> **14.5-oz. can tomato pieces** *(no salt added preferred)* **or 2 cups tomato sauce or 2 cups spaghetti sauce**
> **1 onion, chopped**
> **1 tablespoon chili powder**
> **1½ teaspoons ground cumin seed**
> **1¼ teaspoons salt, to taste** *(RealSalt preferred, p. 269)*

2. Bring just to a boil, reduce heat to simmer for 30 minutes to blend flavors.

1 serving of 4 (about 1½ cups)

Exchanges: 0.5 meat, 3 bread, 1.5 vegetable
299 calories, 14 grams protein (20%), 1 gram fat (3%)
55 grams carbohydrate (77%), 12.5 grams dietary fiber
0 mg. cholesterol, 700 mg. sodium, $.90

VARIATIONS

- ♥ Replace canned beans with **2 cups dry kidney beans**. Cover with **8 cups water** in Crockpot and cook on low overnight or until tender; drain.
- ♥ Add **1 lb.** *Seasoned Ground Turkey* (p. 320)

1 serving of 5 (about 1⅔ cups) with Seasoned Ground Turkey

Exchanges: 3.5 meat, 2.5 bread, 1.25 vegetable
418 calories, 36.5 grams protein (35%), 9.5 grams fat (21%)
45 grams carbohydrate (44%), 10 grams dietary fiber
58 mg. cholesterol, 688 mg. sodium, $1.20

MENU SUGGESTION (606 calories, 27% fat, $1.75):
Chili (meatless)—1 serving (about 1½ cups)
Parmesan greens—2 cups (leafy lettuce, 2 tablespoons Parmesan cheese) with *Soup 'n' Salad Croutons* (p. 361)—¼ cup with *Emilie's Olive Oil Dressing* (p. 372)—½ tablespoon
Carrot sticks—4, orange slices—3
Whole-grain crackers—12 (2 oz.)

COUNTRY CREOLE PEAS 'N' CORN

*A very tasty black-eyed pea dish from **Casseroles** that freezes well. Optional butter gives this dish a yummy flavor, but it is still a family favorite without it and very low in fat!*

AMOUNT: 6 to 8 servings (8-9 cups)

1. Soak 1 to 3 hours in large saucepan:

   2 cups dry black-eyed peas
   8 cups water

2. Bring peas in water to a boil, add seasonings and boil 3 minutes; reduce heat to simmer:

   1 bay leaf (remove before serving)
   1 teaspoon Italian seasoning
   ½ teaspoon rosemary leaves

3. Sauté vegetables in butter (optional for best flavor) or add vegetables uncooked directly to the peas as they cook:

   2 tablespoons unsalted butter (optional)
   1 onion, chopped
   1 green pepper, chopped

4. Continue to cook until peas are almost tender, about 1½ hours. Add more water, if needed.

5. Add remaining ingredients and heat through thoroughly:

   14.5-oz. can stewed tomatoes
   8-oz. can tomato sauce
   ½ stick (¼ cup) butter (optional)
   2 tablespoons honey
   ½ teaspoon salt *(RealSalt preferred, p. 269)*
   1½ cups frozen corn

1 serving of 6 (without optional butter)

Exchanges: 0.5 meat, 2.75 bread, 2 vegetable
300 calories, 16 grams protein (21%), 1 gram fat (3%)
59 grams carbohydrate (76%), 14 grams dietary fiber
0 mg. cholesterol, 604 mg. sodium, $.50

1 serving of 6 with optional butter

Exchanges: 0.5 meat, 2.75 bread, 2.25 fat, 2 vegetable
400 calories, 16 grams protein (16%), 12.5 grams fat (27%)
59 grams carbohydrate (57%), 14 grams dietary fiber
31 mg. cholesterol, 682 mg. sodium, $.60

MENU SUGGESTION (819 calories, 16% fat, $1.35):
Country Creole Peas 'n' Corn—1 serving of 6 with optional butter
Carrot sticks—4, celery sticks—4, cucumber slices—6
Minute Blender Bran Muffins, plain *(p. 356)*—2 with 100% fruit jam—2
   tablespoons

RATATOUILLE

Ratatouille means "easy eggplant." Delicious served over baked potato or brown rice with a whole-grain bread and green salad. Sauté vegetables in oil or butter for richer flavor, or with a little water for extra-low fat.

AMOUNT: 4 servings

1. Sauté onion and garlic in oil or butter, or a little water, until onion is barely tender:

   2 tablespoons olive oil or melted butter (optional)
   1 onion, coarsely chopped
   2 cloves garlic, minced

2. Add and continue cooking until half done:

   1 small eggplant, unpeeled and coarsely chunked
   2 small zucchini, unpeeled and coarsely chunked
   1 green pepper, coarsely chopped

3. Stir in, bring to a boil, lower heat and simmer about 5 minutes:

   2 14.5-oz. cans tomato pieces *(no salt added preferred)*
   ¼ cup minced fresh parsley
   ½ teaspoon basil leaves

4. Blend arrowroot powder or cornstarch into cold water; stir into vegetables, stirring until lightly thickened, about 1-2 minutes:

   2 tablespoons cold water
   4 teaspoons arrowroot powder *(p. 268)* **or cornstarch**

5. Serve with **Parmesan cheese**, if desired.

1 serving of 4 (without optional oil or butter)
Exchanges: 4.25 vegetable
112 calories, 4 grams protein (13%), 1.5 grams fat (10%)
25 grams carbohydrate (77%), 6.5 grams dietary fiber
0 mg. cholesterol, 299 mg. sodium, $.90

1 serving of 4 (with olive oil)
Exchanges: 1.25 fat, 4.25 vegetable
172 calories, 4 grams protein (9%), 8 grams fat (39%)
25 mg. carbohydrate (52%), 6.5 grams dietary fiber
0 mg. cholesterol, 299 mg. sodium, $.95

MENU SUGGESTION (615 calories, 29% fat, $1.55):
Ratatouille—1 serving (made with olive oil)
Baked potato—1 (8 oz.)
Orange tossed salad—2 cups (leafy lettuce, orange chunks, chopped celery) with *Sue's House Dressing* *(p. 373)*—1 tablespoon
Sourdough bread—1 with *Butter Spread* *(p. 371)*—1½ teaspoons

VEGETABLE LASAGNA

A refreshing "no lasagna noodle" lasagna. A great company dish! Note how the fat percentage of the Menu Suggestion below (22%) compares with the fat percentage of this dish (40%).

AMOUNT: 6-8 servings
Bake: 375° for 30 minutes, uncovered

1. Wash, steam about 5 minutes until tender, drain well; chop and set aside:
   1 bunch fresh spinach

2. Sauté vegetables in oil (or in a little water and drain):
   1 tablespoon olive oil (optional)
   $^1/_2$ cup chopped onion
   1 cup diced carrots
   1 clove garlic, minced
   1 cup fresh mushrooms, sliced (add during last minute or two)

3. Blend into sautéed vegetables and simmer 10-15 minutes:
   2 cups tomato sauce or paste or spaghetti sauce
   2.25-oz. can sliced ripe olives, drained
   $1^1/_2$ teaspoons oregano leaves
   1 teaspoon basil leaves

4. While sauce simmers prepare:
   6 cups thin unpeeled zucchini slices (about 3 medium)
   $^1/_2$ cup grated sharp cheddar cheese
   $^1/_2$ cup grated mozzarella cheese

5. Whisk together in a mixing bowl:
   1 cup nonfat or low-fat cottage cheese
   2 eggs
   $^1/_4$ cup Parmesan cheese

6. Make 2 layers of ingredients in lightly greased 9" x 13" pan in this order: zucchini, cottage cheese mixture, spinach, cheeses, sauce.

7. Bake uncovered at 375° for 30 minutes.

1 serving of 6 (includes optional oil)

Exchanges: 1.25 meat, 0.25 milk, 1.25 fat, 3.25 vegetable
230 calories, 19 grams protein (30%), 11 grams fat (40%)
19 grams carbohydrate (30%), 7 grams dietary fiber
88 mg. cholesterol, 852 mg. sodium, $1.05

MENU SUGGESTION (527 calories, 22% fat, $1.90)
Vegetable Lasagna—1 serving of 6; pineapple wedges—2 (5 oz.)
Tossed salad—2 cups, with Sweet Orange Dressing *(p. 373)*
Minute Blender Bran Muffins (p. 356)—1 with 100% fruit jam—$1^1/_2$ teaspoons

BLACK BEAN CHOWDER

A hearty soup with real Mexican flavor! Tastes yummy with grated cheddar cheese (¹/₄ cup) on top. Serve with 2 cups green salad with Sweet Orange Dressing, 2 whole-grain rolls with 2 tablespoons jam (677 calories, 19% fat, $1.70).

AMOUNT: about 14 cups (8 to 10 servings)

1. Bring water to a boil with rice and potatoes; lower heat to a very gentle boil, uncovered, for 30 minutes:

   2¹/₂ quarts water
   ¹/₄ cup long-grain brown rice
   2 medium potatoes, peeled or unpeeled, cubed

2. In separate pan sauté vegetables in oil:

   1 tablespoon olive oil
   1 onion, chopped
   1 red pepper, chopped
   1 green pepper, chopped
   2 cloves garlic, minced

3. After potatoes and rice have cooked the full 30 minutes, add remaining ingredients and continue a very gentle boil about 1 hour until chowder is slightly thickened:

   sautéed vegetables
   15-oz. can black beans, undrained
   15¹/₄-oz. can kidney beans, undrained (*no salt added preferred*)
   16-oz. can vegetarian beans in tomato sauce (*Heinz—pinto beans, available in supermarkets*)
   1¹/₂ cups frozen corn
   1 bay leaf
   1 teaspoon ground cumin seed (*p. 269*)
   1¹/₂ teaspoons chili powder
   3 tablespoons *Sue's "Kitchen Magic"* (*p. 383*)

4. Add salt and pepper to taste. Remove bay leaf.

5. If desired, top each serving with:

   grated cheddar cheese
   chopped cilantro

1 serving of 10 (about 1¹/₂ cups); cheese, cilantro not included

Exchanges: 0.25 meat, 2.5 bread, 0.25 fat, 0.75 vegetable
218 calories, 10 grams protein (18%), 2 grams fat (9%)
42.5 grams carbohydrate (74%), 8.5 grams dietary fiber
0 mg. cholesterol, 952 mg. sodium, $.50

VARIATION

In place of water and *Sue's "Kitchen Magic"* use **2¹/₂ quarts chicken broth** (home-prepared, or *Hain* or *Health Valley* brand, p. 268).

EMILIE'S 10-BEAN SOUP

A terrific economy dish! Actually 9 beans and 1 grain, but we like the sound of 10-Bean. Excellent with green salad, cornbread, French bread, or crackers.

AMOUNT: about 14 cups (serves 10-12 generously)

1. Wash dry beans thoroughly, place in large container, and add enough water to cover beans by 2 inches:

   ¼ cup *each*:

black-eyed peas	split green peas
large lima beans	small lima beans
pinto beans	red beans
navy beans	great northern beans
pearl barley	lentils

2. Let stand 1 hour. Drain, add water, and simmer (covered) for 1½-2 hours until tender:

   2 quarts water

3. Add and simmer 30 minutes to blend flavors:

   1 large onion, chopped
   29-oz. can whole tomatoes or tomato pieces
   1 teaspoon chili powder
   1 clove minced garlic
   juice of 1 lemon
   1 to 2 tablespoons *Sue's "Kitchen Magic,"* **to taste** (p. 383)
   salt and pepper, to taste

1 serving of 10 (about 1½ cups)

Exchanges: 0.5 meat, 2 bread, 0.5 vegetable
187 calories, 11 grams protein (24%), 1 gram fat (4%)
34 grams carbohydrate (73%), 6 grams dietary fiber
0 mg. cholesterol, 680 mg. sodium, $.25

VARIATIONS

♥ In place of the individual dry beans and barley, use a **20-oz. package bean mix** (about 3 cups dry beans). Several bean combinations are available in supermarkets.

♥ Omit step 2; cook beans in 2 quarts water on low overnight in Crockpot until tender.

MENU SUGGESTION (663 calories, 29% fat, $1.10):
Emilie's 10-Bean Soup—1 cup with whole-grain crackers—6
Parmesan greens with croutons/dressing—2 cups *(see menu suggestion, p. 331)*
Pineapple Cornbread (p. 359)—1 piece with *Butter Spread* (p. 371)—1 tablespoon; honey—1 tablespoon

---

CREAMY VEGETABLE CHOWDER

A delectable and colorful soup from **Lunches & Snacks.**

AMOUNT: 9 cups (4 to 6 servings)

1. Melt butter in a large saucepan, add mushrooms and onion; cook until tender, stirring often:

   3 tablespoons melted butter (unsalted preferred)
   4 cups fresh mushrooms, sliced
   1 medium onion, chopped

2. Meanwhile, bring chicken broth to boil in a medium saucepan; add broccoli, bring quickly back to a boil, and let boil for 1 minute; remove from heat:

   2 14.5-oz. cans (or 4 cups) chicken broth (p. 268)
   4 cups fresh broccoli flowers, small pieces

3. Blend flour and seasoning into mushrooms and onion, add milk all at once, stirring until thickened and bubbling; cook 1 minute longer:

   6 tablespoons whole-wheat flour (pastry flour preferred, p. 267) **or unbleached white flour**
   ¹/₂-1 teaspoon salt, to taste (RealSalt preferred, p. 269)
   ¹/₄ teaspoon pepper
   2 13-oz. cans (3¹/₃ cups) evaporated skim milk

4. Stir in and heat through:

   broccoli and chicken broth
   2 cups frozen corn
   4-oz. jar pimiento, drained and chopped

1¹/₂-cup serving

Exchanges: 0.25 meat, 1 milk, 1 bread, 1 fat, 1.75 vegetable
256 calories, 13.5 grams protein (20%), 8 grams fat (26%)
37 grams carbohydrate (54%), 7 grams dietary fiber
23 mg. cholesterol, 520 mg. sodium, $1.60

MENU SUGGESTION (587 calories, 15% fat, $2.20):
Creamy Vegetable Chowder—1¹/₂ cups
Minute Blender Bran Muffins (p. 356)—1 with 100% fruit jam—1 tablespoon
Fresh fruit (¹/₂ apple in wedges, ¹/₂ banana in chunks, 10 grapes)

SWEET 'N' SOUR TOFU STIR-FRY

While tofu does not play a large part in our meals, this recipe is our favorite way to use it in a main dish. Provides high-quality complementary protein with brown rice. Prepare in a wok, if available. Serve immediately.

AMOUNT: 6 to 8 servings

1. Make a **double recipe** *Brown Rice* (p. 312) for ³/₄-1 cup servings.

2. Drain tofu between paper towels on a plate for 30 minutes:
   16-oz. block regular or firm tofu (p. 369)

3. Prepare *Sweet 'n' Sour Sauce* (p. 339).

4. Clean and cut desired **raw vegetables** (p. 341); set aside.

5. In separate bowl whisk together:
   2 eggs
   ¹/₂ cup whole-wheat or whole-wheat pastry flour (p. 367) **or other whole-grain flour**
   ¹/₂ teaspoon salt (optional) (*RealSalt preferred, p. 269*)

6. Cut drained tofu into 1" cubes; fold carefully into egg-flour mixture to coat evenly. Lightly brown coated tofu cubes on both sides in **2 tablespoons olive oil**, or without oil in nonstick pan; remove from pan.

7. Add ¹/₃ **cup water** to pan over medium heat. Add longer cooking vegetables to pan and stir quickly. Cover with lid and cook about 2 minutes, stirring once. Add remaining vegetables, stirring quickly. Cover with lid and cook 2-5 minutes longer until just crisp-tender; stir a time or two.

8. Fold into stir-fried vegetables: **tofu, hot** *Sweet 'n' Sour Sauce*, **pineapple chunks reserved from making sauce.**

1 serving of 6 with 1¹/₂ cups cooked vegetables (rice not included; includes oil in step 6 and salt in step 5)

Exchanges: 1 meat, 0.75 bread, 1 fat, 1.25 fruit, 2.75 vegetable
348 calories, 12 grams protein (13%), 9 grams fat (22%)
59 grams carbohydrate (65%), 5 grams dietary fiber
59 mg. cholesterol, 419 mg. sodium, $1.10

MENU SUGGESTION (763 calories, 14% fat, $1.85):
Sweet 'n' Sour Tofu Stir-Fry—1 serving of 6
Brown Rice (p. 312)—1 cup
Green leaf salad—2 cups (mixed leafy greens with cucumber, chopped parsley, squeeze of lemon juice)
Whole-grain roll—1 with 100% fruit jam—1 tablespoon

SWEET 'N' SOUR SAUCE

A delicious complement to meats such as chicken and meatballs, and stir-fry vegetables. See recipes for Sweet 'n' Sour Tofu Stir-Fry (p. 338) and Cashew Chicken (p. 351). Easy to make! For a smaller recipe, see variation below.

AMOUNT: about 2½ cups (6 to 10 servings)

1. Drain juice into small saucepan and set pineapple chunks aside:

    20-oz. can pineapple chunks, unsweetened (about 1 cup pineapple juice)

2. Blend into juice with wire whisk:

    6-oz. can (¾ cup) pineapple juice, unsweetened
    ⅜ cup plus 2 teaspoons apple cider vinegar
    2½ tablespoons arrowroot powder (p. 268) **or cornstarch**
    1½ tablespoons soy sauce (Kikkoman Lite preferred, p. 269)
    ¼ cup plus 1 tablespoon honey
    ⅜ teaspoon ground ginger

3. Bring to a boil over medium heat, whisking constantly until thickened, about 1 minute.

4. Fold hot sauce and reserved pineapple chunks into desired meat or stir-fry vegetable recipe.

1 serving of 6 (scant ½ cup sauce, ¼ cup pineapple chunks)

Exchanges: 0.25 bread, 1.25 fruit
146 calories, 37 grams carbohydrate (97%)
0 mg. cholesterol, 159 mg. sodium, $.35.

VARIATION
For a smaller sauce recipe (1½ cups) use the following amounts:
6-oz. can (¾ cup) pineapple juice, unsweetened
⅓ cup apple cider vinegar
2 tablespoons arrowroot powder (p. 268) **or cornstarch**
1 tablespoon soy sauce (Kikkoman Lite preferred, p. 269)
¼ cup honey
½ teaspoon ground ginger
1 cup fresh pineapple chunks (optional)

1 serving of 6 (about ¼ cup sauce with ¼ cup fresh pineapple)

Exchanges: 0.25 bread, 0.5 fruit
93 calories, 24 grams carbohydrate (96%), 0.5 gram dietary fiber
0 mg. cholesterol, 101 mg. sodium, $.20

MARINATED TOFU STIR-FRY

Tofu is the easily digestible portion of soybeans mixed with water and coagulated into curds with natural minerals. It is a good source of complementary protein to grain, a good calcium source, and contains no cholesterol or lactose. Tofu is 39% fat in calories, three times higher in unsaturated than saturated fat. To store fresh tofu, drain off liquid and cover with fresh water; refrigerate. Change water every 2 days and use within 2 weeks. Tofu packaged for long-term storage is also available.

AMOUNT: 6 servings

1. Drain tofu between paper towels on plate for 30 minutes:

     16-oz. block regular or firm tofu (p. 269)

2. Meanwhile, blend together for marinade:

     1/2 cup soy sauce Kikkoman Lite preferred, p. 269
     3 tablespoons lemon juice (fresh preferred)
     1 teaspoon ground ginger
     1/8 teaspoon garlic powder

3. Cut tofu into 1" cubes and place in marinade for 1 hour or longer.

4. Make a **double recipe Brown Rice** (p. 312) for 1-cup servings.

5. Clean and cut vegetables for stir-fry (p. 341, step 1)

6. Brown **marinated tofu cubes** in:

     1 tablespoon olive oil or melted butter (unsalted preferred)

7. Stir-fry the vegetables in **1/3 cup water** (p. 341, step 2)**; fold in tofu cubes.**

1 serving of 6 with 1 1/2 cups cooked vegetables (rice not included)

Exchanges: 0.5 meat, 0.25 bread, 0.5 fat, 2.75 vegetable
143 calories, 8.5 grams protein (22%), 4.5 grams fat (27%)
19.5 grams carbohydrate (51%), 3.5 grams dietary fiber
0 mg. cholesterol, 77 mg. sodium, $.70

VARIATIONS
Add **cashews or almonds.**

MENU SUGGESTION (655 calories, 16% fat, $1.50):
Marinated Tofu Stir-Fry—1 serving; *Brown Rice* (p. 312)—1 cup
Green leaf salad—2 cups (mixed leafy greens with cucumber, chopped parsley) with *Sue's House Dressing* (p. 373)—1 tablespoon
Minute Blender Bran Muffins (p. 356)—1 with 100% fruit jam—1 tablespoon

---

STIR-FRY VEGETABLES

Vegetables that lend themselves to diagonal cutting add to the beauty of stir-fry dishes and facilitate the speed of cooking. Cut them thinly to speed cooking. Serve alone with dash of soy sauce or with Sweet 'n' Sour Sauce (p. 339), with Sweet 'n' Sour Tofu Stir-Fry (p. 338), with Marinated Tofu Stir-Fry (p. 340), or add cooked beef or chicken strips, and/or cashews, as desired. Serve immediately over brown rice. Have entire meal prepared and table set before you start to stir-fry the vegetables. Best prepared in a wok.

AMOUNT: prepare 1-1¹/₂ cups cooked vegetables per serving
  Note: Volume of raw vegetables required will depend on what vegetables you choose. The more vegetables used that cook down considerably (such as leafy greens, bean sprouts, onion, and cabbage), the more volume of raw vegetables you will need for 1-1¹/₂ cups cooked.

1. Clean and cut desired selection of vegetables thinly, placing the shorter cooking vegetables in the bottom of a large bowl with the longer cooking ones on top in about the following order (shorter cooking vegetables listed first), or arrange separately on a plate:

   leafy greens such as spinach or chard—finely shredded
   water chestnuts—drained, rinsed, sliced
   mushrooms—sliced
   zucchini, yellow squash slices—cut diagonally
   bean sprouts—fresh
   green onion—chopped
   cabbage, bok choy, napa cabbage, red—shredded
   bell pepper strips (green, red, yellow)
   broccoli—flowers in small pieces, stalks cut diagonally
   cauliflower—small flowers
   red, brown, or yellow onion—cut in rings
   celery—cut diagonally
   carrot slices—cut diagonally
   green beans—cut diagonally

2. Add ¹/₃ **cup water or 1 tablespoon olive oil** to hot pan over medium-high heat. Add longer-cooking vegetables; stir quickly. Cover and cook about 2 minutes, stirring once. Add shorter-cooking vegetables; stir quickly. Cover and cook 2-5 minutes longer until just crisp-tender; stir a time or two.

1 cup cooked vegetables (average of 12 cooked vegetables, no oil)

Exchanges: 0.25 fat (with oil only), 1.75 vegetable
46 calories, 2 grams protein (18%), less than 0.5 gram fat (4%)
10 grams carbohydrate (78%), 2.5 grams dietary fiber
0 mg. cholesterol, 36 mg. sodium, $.30

TOFU SCRAMBLE

A tasty low-cholesterol alternative to scrambled eggs from **Breakfasts!** *Even if you do eat scrambled eggs, try this for variety. Don't expect it to look like scrambled eggs, however.*

AMOUNT: 4 servings

1. Drain tofu thoroughly for 30 minutes between paper towels on a large dinner plate:

    16-oz. block firm or regular tofu *(p. 269)*

2. Mash tofu coarsely with a fork on a clean, dry plate; put crumbled tofu in a mixing bowl and blend in:

    ¼ cup Bragg Liquid Aminos *(see note below)* **or 2 tablespoons soy sauce** *(Kikkoman Lite preferred, p. 269)*
    ½ teaspoon dry mustard

3. Fold in:

    4 fresh mushrooms, sliced
    1 green onion, chopped
    1 canned green chile, finely diced *(p. 268)*

4. Heat frying pan over moderate heat; add and coat bottom of pan with:

    1 tablespoon olive oil or butter (do not allow to burn)

5. Add tofu mixture. Cover and cook over medium heat about 15 minutes until slightly set.

6. Top with:

    ½ cup grated cheddar, Jack, or mozzarella cheese
    garnish of paprika

7. Serve as desired with **salsa, catsup, barbecue sauce**.

1 serving of 4 (does not include sauce topping in step 7)

Exchanges: 1.5 meat, 0.25 bread, 1.25 fat, 0.5 vegetable
177 calories, 12 grams protein (28%), 12 grams fat (61%)
5 grams carbohydrate (12%), 0.5 gram dietary fiber
15 mg. cholesterol, 111 mg. sodium, $.94

MENU SUGGESTION (435 calories, 28% fat, $1.60)
Cantaloupe—¼ medium
Tofu Scramble—1 serving
Whole-grain toast—2 slices with 100% fruit jam—1 tablespoon
Herb tea

Bragg Liquid Aminos is a liquid similar to soy sauce derived from fermented soybeans, but has no added salt. It is a tasty seasoning, high in protein. Purchase at a health-food store.

LITTLE COTTAGE ENCHILADAS

*The green sauce tingles with a hot zap. One husband decided that "Eating Better" was worth trying after eating this recipe from **Main Dishes**! For children you may want to fewer less chiles.*

AMOUNT: 4 servings
Bake: 400° for 15-20 minutes, uncovered

1. Set aside 1 cup of the grated cheese and combine the rest with remaining ingredients:

   2 cups grated cheddar cheese
   1 cup low-fat or nonfat cottage cheese
   ¹/₂ teaspoon thyme leaves
   ¹/₂ teaspoon marjoram leaves
   ¹/₂ teaspoon oregano leaves

2. For green sauce, liquify first 3 ingredients in blender; then simmer for 3 minutes in the melted butter:

   ¹/₂ cup water
   3 large outer leaves romaine lettuce
   4-oz. can diced chiles, drained
   1 tablespoon melted butter *(unsalted preferred)*

3. Pour ²/₃ of the sauce in baking dish and distribute evenly over the bottom (use a baking dish in which 6 rolled and filled tortillas will fit in a single layer).

4. Heat tortillas in ungreased frying pan over moderate heat:

   6 stoneground corn tortillas *(p. 267)*

5. Fill each tortilla with ¹/₃-cup cheese mixture, roll up, and place in baking dish with edges tucked underneath. Pour remaining sauce over tortillas and top with:

   remaining cup grated cheddar cheese

6. Bake uncovered at 400° for 15-20 minutes until heated through and cheese melts.

1 serving of 4 (1¹/₂ enchiladas)

Exchanges: 2 meat, 0.5 milk, 1 bread, 3 fat, 0.5 vegetable
391 calories, 24 grams protein (25%), 23 grams fat (54%)
21 grams carbohydrate (21%), 3 grams dietary fiber
72 mg. cholesterol, 594 mg. sodium, $1.10

MENU SUGGESTION (711 calories, 31% fat, $1.55)
Little Cottage Enchiladas—1 serving (1¹/₂ enchiladas)
Brown Rice *(p. 312)*—³/₄ cup; cooked carrots—³/₄ cup
Salad: orange slices—3, fresh pineapple wedges—2 (5 oz.), and
   cucumber slices—3, on loose leaf lettuce with *Sweet Lite Dressing* *(p. 373)*—1 tablespoon

---

NOODLE PARMESAN SUPREME

*A meatless dish from **Casseroles** that freezes well if light sour cream is substituted for yogurt in step 3. Experiment with different kinds of whole-grain noodles besides whole-wheat from the health-food store such as spinach or artichoke pasta, spelt, or Kamut. Kamut noodles are especially light and highest of the grains in protein and minerals. If you can find Kamut noodles, you will undoubtedly like them best!*

AMOUNT: 4 servings

1. To cook pasta, bring water to a boil with salt and oil, add noodles, and cook just until tender, according to time given on package directions; add broccoli and zucchini to noodles during the last minute; drain:

   4 quarts boiling water
   $1/4$ teaspoon salt *(RealSalt preferred, p. 269)*
   1 teaspoon olive oil
   8 oz. whole-grain noodles *(p. 267)*
   1 cup broccoli flowerets
   1 cup chopped, unpeeled zucchini (1 small)

2. Sauté almonds and garlic in butter (optional for flavor):

   1 tablespoon melted unsalted butter (optional)
   $1/4$ cup almonds, slivered, sliced, or chopped
   2 cloves garlic, minced

3. Blend together and stir into almonds and garlic:

   1 cup nonfat yogurt (or $1/2$-1 cup light sour cream)
   $1/2$ cup light sour cream
   2 tablespoons whole-wheat or whole-wheat pastry flour *(preferred, p. 267)* **or unbleached white flour**
   $1/2$ cup Parmesan cheese
   $1/2$ teaspoon salt, to taste *(RealSalt preferred, p. 269)*

4. Fold in drained noodles and vegetables; heat through over moderately low heat until hot throughout but do not let the sauce boil (may also be heated in casserole dish in the oven).

1 serving of 4 (with optional butter, nonfat yogurt in step 3)

Exchanges: 1.5 meat, 0.5 milk, 2.75 bread, 2.25 fat, 0.5 vegetable
438 calories, 21.5 grams protein (19%), 18.5 grams fat (37%)
50 grams carbohydrate (44%), 8.5 grams dietary fiber
27 mg. cholesterol, 662 mg. sodium, $1.00

MENU SUGGESTION (731 calories, 25% fat, $1.75)
Noodle Parmesan Supreme—1 serving
Tossed salad—2 cups (leafy lettuce, red cabbage, celery, carrot, tomato, radishes) with *Sweet Orange Dressing* (p. 373)
Minute Blender Bran Muffins, raisin (p. 356)—1 with 100% fruit jam— 1 tablespoon

---

TUNA NOODLE YUMMY

One of our favorite recipes from **Main Dishes***, this is a variation of Noodle Parmesan Supreme (p. 344). Will freeze well if light sour cream is substituted for the yogurt in step 3. Tuna fish contains omega-3 fatty acids that may lower heart disease risk.*

AMOUNT: 6 servings

1. Follow step 1 for *Noodle Parmesan Supreme (p. 344)* to cook the noodles, omitting broccoli and zucchini.

2. Meanwhile, in large saucepan lightly cook onion and celery in a little water; drain:

   ¹/₂ onion, chopped
   ¹/₂ cup celery (1 large rib), chopped

3. Fold together in saucepan with the cooked celery and onion:

   1 cup nonfat yogurt (or ¹/₂-1 cup light sour cream)
   ¹/₂ cup light sour cream
   2 tablespoons whole-wheat or whole-wheat pastry flour *(preferred, p. 267)***, or unbleached white flour**
   ¹/₃ cup Parmesan cheese
   6.25-oz. can water pack tuna *(50% salt reduced preferred)* **sprinkled with 1 teaspoon lemon juice**
   ¹/₂ cup frozen green peas
   ¹/₂ teaspoon salt, to taste *(RealSalt preferred, p. 269)*
   cooked, drained noodles

4. Heat over moderately low heat until hot throughout but do not let the sauce boil (may also be heated in casserole dish in the oven).

1 serving of 6 (with nonfat yogurt in step 3)

Exchanges: 1.25 meat, 0.25 milk, 2 bread, 0.5 fat, 0.25 vegetable
283 calories, 19.5 grams protein (27%), 7.5 grams fat (24%)
36 grams carbohydrate (49%), 5 grams dietary fiber
29 mg. cholesterol, 492 mg. sodium, $.85

VARIATION

♥ Add the sautéed almonds and garlic (step 2, *p. 344*). Increase Parmesan cheese to ¹/₂ cup.

MENU SUGGESTION (672 calories, 23% fat, $1.80)
Tuna Noodle Yummy—1 serving; cooked carrots—³/₄ cup
Salad: tomato slices—3, cucumber slices—6 on leafy lettuce with
   Emilie's Olive Oil Dressing (p. 372)—1 tablespoon
Whole-grain roll—1¹/₂ with 100% fruit jam—1¹/₂ tablespoons

LEMON BAKED FISH

A simple but delicious recipe for any lean fish. Purchase a 6-oz. fish fillet or 8-oz. steak per serving of halibut, cod, sole, flounder, mahimahi, ocean perch, pollock, tilapia, sea bass, orange roughy, whiting, red snapper, or any other lean fish.

AMOUNT: 4 servings
Bake: 350° for 20-30 minutes, uncovered

1. Place in bottom of baking pan and melt at low heat in oven:

   ¼ **cup (½ stick) butter** *(unsalted preferred)*

2. Remove pan from oven and turn oven to 350° to preheat; place fish in single layer in buttered pan:

   1½ lbs. fish fillets or 2 lbs. fish steaks

3. Spoon some of the melted butter over top of fish.

4. Squeeze over the top:

   juice of 1 lemon (or about 4 teaspoons)

5. Lightly sprinkle with:

   1¼ teaspoons *Sue's Fish Herb Seasoning* (p. 347)

6. Bake uncovered for 20-30 minutes at 350° until fish is tender, basting 1 or 2 times. Fish is done when it flakes easily with a fork and the translucent flesh has turned opaque. Do not overcook!

1 serving of 4 (6-oz. fillet of sole)

Exchanges: 2.75 meat, 1.25 fat
213 calories, 34 grams protein (66%), 7.5 grams fat (33%)
0.5 gram carbohydrate (1%)
133 mg. cholesterol, 203 mg. sodium, $1.70

VARIATIONS

♥ Top fish with ½ small onion, thinly sliced.
♥ In place of *Sue's Fish Herb Seasoning*, lightly sprinkle fish with paprika, salt to taste, fresh minced or dried parsley.
♥ For reduced fat: Omit butter. Lay fish in pan coated with olive oil nonstick spray. Add a couple tablespoons of water. Cover tightly to bake; baste 2 or 3 times.

MENU SUGGESTION (517 calories, 26% fat, $2.40)
Lemon Baked Fish—1 serving with *Tartar Sauce* (p. 347)—2 tablespoons
Brown Rice Pilaf (p. 313)—1 serving (about ¾ cup)
Broccoli-Carrot Medley (p. 363)—1 serving, or frozen peas
Sliced tomatoes—3 with sliced cucumber—6, on leafy greens

TARTAR SAUCE

Everyone wants tartar sauce with fish! Try this blend of nonfat yogurt with a little mayonnaise for a tasty lower-fat version!

AMOUNT: scant ¹/₂ cup (serves 4)

Blend thoroughly with a wire whisk:

¹/₃ cup plain nonfat yogurt
1 tablespoon mayonnaise *(p. 269)*
1 tablespoon sweet pickle relish
1¹/₂ teaspoons lemon juice
¹/₂ teaspoon mustard *(no salt added preferred, p. 269)*
¹/₈ teaspoon dill weed
¹/₈ teaspoon garlic powder

1 scant tablespoon

Exchanges: 0.25 fat
21 calories, 0.5 gram protein (11%), 1.5 grams fat (67%)
1 gram carbohydrate (22%)
0 mg. cholesterol, 29 mg. sodium, $.05

SUE'S FISH HERB SEASONING

A tasty seasoning for any lean fish such as halibut, cod, sole, flounder, mahimahi, ocean perch, pollock, tilapia, sea bass, orange roughy, whiting, red snapper.

³/₈ cup (seasons 12-20 lbs. fish)

Blend thoroughly and store in tightly covered container in refrigerator or freezer; season fish with it, to taste:

1 tablespoon onion powder
1 tablespoon dill weed
1 tablespoon garlic powder
1 tablespoon thyme leaves, crushed
1 tablespoon paprika
1 tablespoon dried parsley flakes

Approximate Cost: $1.80

LEMON BAKED SALMON

Good for any fat fish such as bluefish, herring, mackerel, pompano, whitefish, salmon, mullet, sablefish. Salmon contains omega-3 fatty acids that may lower heart disease risk, so don't disparage the high fat content of salmon!

AMOUNT: 4 to 6 servings
Bake: 350° for 20-30 minutes, uncovered

1. Place in bottom of baking pan and melt at low heat in oven:

   1 tablespoon butter *(unsalted preferred)*

2. Remove pan from oven and turn oven to 350° to preheat; lay steaks evenly in pan in melted butter and top evenly with remaining ingredients:

   2 lbs. salmon steaks
   juice of ¹/₂-1 lemon (or 3-4 teaspoons)
   ¹/₈ teaspoon salt (optional) *(RealSalt preferred, p. 269)*
   paprika
   fresh minced or dried parsley flakes

3. Bake uncovered at 350° for 20-30 minutes, basting 1 or 2 times. Fish is done when it flakes easily with a fork and the translucent flesh has turned opaque. Do not overcook!

1 serving of 6 (about 5 oz.)

Exchanges: 4 meat, 0.5 fat
267 calories, 37.5 grams protein (60%), 11 grams fat (39%)
112 mg. cholesterol, 143 mg. sodium, $2.20

MENU SUGGESTION (793 calories, 23% fat, $3.50)
Lemon Baked Salmon—1 serving of 6 (5 oz.)
Tartar Sauce (p. 347)—2 tablespoons
Broccoli, Orange & Fig Salad (p. 360)—1 serving
Minute Blender Bran Muffins (p. 356)—1 with 100% fruit jam—1 table-spoon

---

ALMOND TUNA SALAD

A very filling, lovely to look at, refreshing salad for a summer evening meal. Tuna fish contains omega-3 fatty acids that may lower heart disease risk.

AMOUNT: 2 servings

1. Mix together:

   6.25-oz. can water-packed tuna, well drained (salt reduced preferred)
   ¼ cup nonfat plain yogurt
   2 tablespoons mayonnaise (p. 269)
   2 teaspoons lemon juice (fresh preferred)
   1 rib celery, chopped
   1 slice onion, chopped
   ⅓ cup chopped or slivered almonds

2. Arrange on each individual salad plate in the following order:

   leaf of leafy green lettuce
   2 cups broken leafy and iceberg lettuce
   1 tomato, cut almost through in wedges to form a tomato "flower"
   half the tuna mixture mounded in center of tomato "flower"
   garnish paprika on tuna mixture
   ripe olive in center of tuna mixture

3. Garnish with **parsley sprigs**.

1 serving

Exchanges: 2.25 meat, 0.25 milk, 0.25 bread, 4.5 fat, 2.25 vegetable
423 calories, 29 grams protein (26%), 27 grams fat (56%)
20 grams carbohydrate (18%), 6 grams dietary fiber
59 mg. cholesterol, 399 mg. sodium, $1.95

MENU SUGGESTION (897 calories, 30% fat, $3.25)
Almond Tuna Salad—1 serving
Carrot sticks—4, cucumber slices—6
Whole-grain rolls—2 with 100% fruit jam—2 tablespoons
Fresh peach, sliced—1 with honey yogurt topping (½ cup nonfat plain yogurt with 1½ teaspoons honey)

BAKED PARMESAN CHICKEN

*Our gourmet favorite from **Main Dishes** for company and banquets! Note the dramatic difference in the fat content of the reduced-fat version, but note, too, the menu percentage of fat with the higher-fat version.*

AMOUNT: 6 servings (5.3 oz. each)
Bake: 350° for 1 hour, uncovered

1. Melt butter in baking pan at about 250°:
   ¹/₂ cup (1 stick) butter *(unsalted preferred)*

2. Meanwhile, blend together in blender until small bread crumbs are formed:
   1 slice whole-wheat bread *(p. 267)* **or amount needed to make about 1 cup soft crumbs, not packed**
   2 or 3 sprigs parsley to make about ¹/₄ cup minced
   ¹/₂ cup Parmesan cheese
   ¹/₈ teaspoon salt *(RealSalt preferred, p. 269)*
   ¹/₈ teaspoon garlic powder

3. Remove visible fat from chicken:
   2 lbs. skinless, boneless chicken breast pieces

4. Coat pieces of chicken in melted butter in pan, then coat with crumb mixture; lay single layer in remaining butter in pan.

5. Garnish with **paprika** and bake uncovered at 350° until tender, about 1 hour; basted 2 or 3 times during baking. Cover with foil if chicken begins to brown too much before done.

1 serving
___
4.5 meat, 0.25 bread, 3 fat
411 calories, 48 grams protein (47%), 22.5 grams fat (50%)
3 grams carbohydrate (3%), 0.5 gram dietary fiber
163 mg. cholesterol, 296 mg. sodium, $1.65

REDUCED FAT VARIATION

♥ Reduce to **3 tablespoons Parmesan cheese.**

♥ Omit butter; bake in pan coated with olive oil nonstick spray.

♥ Dip chicken pieces in nonfat milk, as needed, in place of butter.

1 serving Reduced Fat Variation
___
4 meat, 0.25 bread
265 calories, 46.5 grams protein (21%), 6 grams fat (21%)
4 grams carbohydrate (6%), 0.5 gram dietary fiber
119 mg. cholesterol, 216 mg. sodium, $1.50

MENU SUGGESTION (833 calories, 30% fat, $2.45)
Baked Parmesan Chicken (not Reduced Fat Variation)—1 serving
Brown Rice Pilaf (p. 313)—³/₄ cup; broccoli (p. 362)—³/₄ cup
Pineapple Sunshine Mold—no nuts (p. 374)—1 serving on greens
Whole-grain roll—1 with 100% fruit jam—1 tablespoon

CASHEW CHICKEN

With Sweet 'n' Sour Sauce this is a very colorful, savory dish! Serve over brown rice or whole-grain noodles.

AMOUNT: 4 to 6 servings

1. Cook whole-grain noodles (for 1-cup servings use 12 oz. for 4, 16 oz. for 6; follow package directions, adding **1 teaspoon olive oil** and **¼ teaspoon salt** to the water; or cook *Brown Rice* (p. 312). (Double the recipe for 6 1-cup servings).

2. Skin chicken and cut into bite-sized chunks; cover with water and bring to a boil. Reduce heat to a very gentle boil for about 30 minutes or until chicken is tender:

   1 lb. boneless chicken breast to make 2 cups chicken

3. Prepare *Sweet 'n' Sour Sauce* (p. 339), using Variation for the smaller recipe (for the fresh pineapple, see step 5 below).

3. Sauté vegetables in a little water or oil until crisp-tender, adding peas or spinach and red pepper the last minute or two of cooking (drain any water):

   1 tablespoon olive oil (optional)
   2 cups celery, sliced thinly on diagonal
   1 medium onion, sliced
   ½ cup fresh or frozen green peas or 1 head lightly steamed, chopped spinach
   1 red bell pepper cut in strips or 2-oz. jar pimiento, drained

5. Fold into sautéed vegetables and heat thoroughly:

   cooked chicken
   ½ cup unsalted roasted cashews
   1 cup fresh pineapple chunks
   Sweet 'n' Sour Sauce

1 serving of 6 (noodles or rice not included)

Exchanges: 1.5 meat, 0.5 bread, 1 fat, 0.75 fruit, 1 vegetable
282 calories, 18 grams protein (25%), 8.5 grams fat (26%)
36 grams carbohydrate (49%), 3.5 grams dietary fiber
38 mg. cholesterol, 188 mg. sodium, $1.45

MENU SUGGESTION (653 calories, 24% fat, $2.45)
Cashew Chicken—1 serving of 6
Cooked whole-grain noodles—1 cup
Green leaf salad—2 cups (mixed leafy greens with cucumber, chopped parsley, squeeze of lemon juice)

RAGOUT

"Ragoo," but my mother who made this easy down-home dish with bacon and ground beef called it "Rag-OUT." It was a family favorite. Now we do it without the bacon and use seasoned ground turkey. Good served with catsup!

AMOUNT: 4 to 6 servings

1. In a wok or pot that will hold all the ingredients, brown:

   1 lb. *Seasoned Ground Turkey* (p. 320)

2. Layer over browned turkey in order given:

   1 large onion, sliced
   6 medium carrots, thinly sliced
   4 medium potatoes, thinly sliced (unpeeled preferred)
   $^1/_2$-1 cup water, or as needed

3. Season to taste with **salt and pepper**, cover tightly; simmer until vegetables are tender, about 30 minutes.

1 serving of 4 (with $^1/_4$ teaspoon salt, $^1/_8$ teaspoon pepper used in recipe)

Exchanges: 3.5 meat, 0.75 bread, 2.75 vegetable
348 calories, 35 grams protein (39%), 11 grams fat (28%)
30 grams carbohydrate (33%), 7.5 grams dietary fiber
72 mg. cholesterol, 337 mg. sodium, $.80

VARIATIONS

Add during last 8-10 minutes of cooking, as desired: **10 oz. (2 cups) frozen cut green beans, green peas, or corn.**

MENU SUGGESTION (602 calories, 27% fat, $1.40)
Ragout—1 serving with catsup—2 tablespoons
Corn on cob—1 5" ear with *Butter Spread* (p. 371)—1$^1/_2$ teaspoons
Coleslaw—1 cup ($^3/_4$ cup cabbage, $^1/_4$ cup crushed pineapple) with
  Sweet Lite Dressing (p. 373)—1 tablespoon

EGG REAL FOOL! SANDWICH

*Some people are sure the tofu filling tastes just like egg. Try the filling on pita bread as well as sandwich bread. Filling keeps in refrigerator for several days. This recipe comes from the Children's Cookbook section of **Lunches & Snacks**. Instructions are written for children.*

AMOUNT: 3 cups filling

1. *Open* **16-oz. block regular or firm tofu** and *drain* off all the liquid. Place block of tofu between 2 layers of paper towel on a dinner plate for at least 30 minutes to remove more moisture.

2. *Tofu Salad Spread:* Remove wet paper towel, place tofu on a dry plate, and *mash* it with a fork. Place it in a mixing bowl and thoroughly *mix* in the remaining ingredients:

   16 oz. (2 cups) tofu, well drained, mashed
   ¹/₂ cup finely chopped onion
   2 ribs finely chopped celery
   ¹/₄ cup finely chopped green pepper
   ¹/₄ cup mayonnaise (p. 269) (half may be yogurt)
   1 to 2 tablespoons apple cider vinegar, to taste
   2 teaspoons mustard
   ¹/₂ teaspoon garlic powder
   ¹/₄ teaspoon tumeric (for color; a spice at supermarkets)

3. *Spread* on **whole-grain bread** to make some delicious sandwiches! Choose a different shape for the bread, for fun. Add **dark leafy green lettuce** and **sliced tomatoes or avocado**, if desired.

VARIATION
Serve *Tofu Salad Spread* in pita bread with desired veggies.

¹/₃ cup Tofu Salad Spread only

Exchanges: 0.5 meat, 1 fat, 0.25 vegetable
88 calories, 4 grams protein (17%), 6.5 grams fat (69%)
3 grams carbohydrate (14%), 0.5 gram dietary fiber
2 mg. cholesterol, 53 mg. sodium, $.25

MENU SUGGESTION (411 calories, 29% fat, $.95)
Egg Real Fool! Sandwich:
   2 slices whole-grain bread with ¹/₃ cup *Tofu Salad Spread*, leafy lettuce, ¹/₂ medium tomato in slices, ¹/₆ medium avocado in slices
Carrot sticks—4
Apple—1 medium

GOLDEN WAFFLES/PANCAKES

So you don't have time to make waffles or pancakes for breakfast? Why not have them for an easy and economical dinner! This recipe makes amazingly light waffles when beaten egg whites are added (see Variation). For waffles we like our batter a little on the thin side. If you are not accustomed to keeping fresh buttermilk on hand, powdered buttermilk can be purchased at a health-food store. Store it in the refrigerator and use 3-4 tablespoons powder per 1 cup water.

AMOUNT: 4 to 6 servings

1. Blend together dry ingredients:

   1¹/₂ cups whole-wheat pastry or whole-wheat flour
   1¹/₂ cups stoneground cornmeal *(p. 267)*
   1 tablespoon baking powder *(low sodium or Rumford, p. 268)*
   1 teaspoon salt *(RealSalt preferred, p. 269)*

2. Mix into dry ingredients:

   2¹/₄ cups buttermilk, as desired for consistency
   4 eggs
   3 tablespoons olive oil or melted butter (optional for crispness)
   1¹/₂ teaspoons vanilla

3. Spray hot waffle iron or pancake griddle well with olive oil nonstick spray if oil or butter is not added to batter. Bake 1¹/₂-3 minutes in waffle iron (depends on your iron).

1 serving of 6 with 1% fat buttermilk (includes optional oil)

Exchanges: 0.75 meat, 0.5 milk, 3.25 bread, 1.75 fat
386 calories, 13 grams protein (13%), 13 grams fat (30%)
57 grams carbohydrate (57%), 8 grams dietary fiber
145 mg. cholesterol, 500 mg. sodium, $.55

VARIATIONS

♥ For lighter waffles or pancakes, separate the eggs, beat egg whites until stiff, but not dry, and fold into batter last.

♥ Add chopped nuts to batter or sprinkle over top of each waffle just before closing the waffle iron lid. Try pecans or sunflower seeds.

> **MENU SUGGESTION** (700 calories, 19% fat, $1.45):
> *Golden Waffles (with oil added)*—1 serving of 6
> Applesauce—¹/₂ cup
> Maple syrup—2 tablespoons
> Low-fat vanilla yogurt—¹/₂ cup
> Orange sections—¹/₂ orange

5-MINUTE BLENDER WAFFLES

Our "million-dollar" candidate for the "perfect recipe" from **Breakfasts**—*truly amazing! So fast and so light! Put the whole grain,* unground and uncooked *into the blender with the liquid ingredients. The blender will "make" it into flour. Do not use an old blender with dull blades or worn motor. Use a blender that will grind ice cubes. An Osterizer 10-speed works well.*

AMOUNT: 5 or 6 7" waffles (serves 4)

1. Put into the blender and blend at high speed for 3-4 minutes:

    1¹/₂-1³/₄ cups buttermilk (we like it thinner) *(p. 268)*
    1 egg or 2 egg whites
    2 tablespoons olive oil (optional for crispness)
    1 teaspoon vanilla extract
    1 cup millet *(p. 267)* **or brown rice** (do not use instant)
    ¹/₂ cup quick or regular rolled oats, uncooked

2. Add and blend briefly to mix in:

    2 teaspoons baking powder (low sodium or Rumford, p. 268)
    1 teaspoon salt *(RealSalt preferred, p. 269)*
    ¹/₂ teaspoon baking soda

3. Pour from blender into hot waffle iron, not quite full; bake about 1¹/₂-3 minutes until lightly golden (baking time depends on your waffle iron).

1 waffle of 6 with 1% fat buttermilk (includes olive oil)

Exchanges: 0.25 meat, 0.5 milk, 2.25 bread, 1 fat
235 calories, 8.5 grams protein (14%), 7.5 grams fat (28%)
37 grams carbohydrate (59%), 2 grams dietary fiber
38 mg. cholesterol, 511 mg. sodium, $.35

GRAIN VARIATIONS

♥ Try one of the following grain combinations:
    ¹/₂ cup each: millet, brown rice, oats
    1 cup Kamut, ¹/₂ cup oats
    ¹/₂ cup each millet, brown rice, ¹/₄ cup each oats, kasha
    ³/₄ cup whole wheat, ³/₄ cup dry corn

♥ To make recipe with flour in place of oats and grain, use **2 cups flour**. Blend ingredients in mixing bowl with wire whisk.

PANCAKES—Use a little less buttermilk for a thicker batter.

> **MENU SUGGESTION** (769 calories, 20% fat, $1.85):
> *5-Minute Blender Waffles*—2
> *Alice's Fruit Soup (p. 367)*—1 cup with ¹/₂ banana, sliced
> Low-fat vanilla yogurt—¹/₂ cup

MINUTE BLENDER BRAN MUFFINS

*Our classic family favorite from which all our other muffin recipes in the **Eating Better Cookbooks** have been developed. For many years we made these the traditional way—in a mixing bowl with flour (see the Variation below). Now that we have discovered "blender batter baking" (blending the fresh whole grain with the liquids in the blender) we are using and liking it more and more! Now you can get fresh whole grains without a grain mill! (Be sure to see comments on 5-Minute Blender Waffles, p. 355).*

AMOUNT: 10 large muffins
Bake: 350° for 20 minutes

1. Preheat oven. Grease or spray muffin pan (if two average-size 12-cup muffin pans available, use the pan with deeper cups).

2. Thoroughly stir water into bran in a *large* mixing bowl; let stand 5 minutes to soften bran:
    1½ cups unprocessed wheat bran *(p. 267)*
    ½ cup boiling hot water

3. *Optional:* Stir into the moistened bran as desired:
    ½ cup raisins (softened in water 5 minutes, drained)
    ½ cup walnuts

4. Place in blender in order given; blend on high speed 3-4 minutes:
    1 cup buttermilk *(p. 268)* **or apple juice**
    1 egg or 2 egg whites
    ⅓ cup honey (warm 20 seconds in microwave, if needed to pour)
    1 cup whole-wheat pastry grain (not flour) *(p. 270)*

5. Blend in briefly just to mix in:
    1¼ teaspoons baking soda
    1 teaspoon salt *(RealSalt preferred, p. 269)*

6. Pour batter into bran mixture; fold in just until mixed.

7. Evenly fill 10 muffin cups, leaving the 2 center ones empty. Fill the center cups with water (if you use muffin papers you will need to fill all 12 of the cups with batter).

8. Bake at 350° for 20 minutes. Cool muffins in pan for 5-10 minutes for easy removal (gently tug on side of each muffin).

VARIATION IN PROCEDURE

To make the standard way, omit the grain from step 4. Blend **1½ cups whole-wheat pastry flour** with **soda and salt** (see step 5). Whisk the bran mixture into the blended liquid ingredients in large mixing bowl. Fold in the dry ingredients just until mixed. Fold in raisins and/or walnuts, as desired.

1 plain muffin of 10 with 1% fat buttermilk (no raisins or walnuts)

Exchanges: 0.25 milk, 1.25 bread
144 calories, 5 grams protein (10%), 1.5 grams fat (9%)
33 grams carbohydrate (67%), 5 grams dietary fiber
22 mg. cholesterol, 350 mg. sodium, $.15

1 raisin muffin of 10 with 1% fat buttermilk

Exchanges: 0.25 milk, 1.25 bread, 0.25 fruit
166 calories, 5 grams protein (9%), 1.5 grams fat (8%)
36 grams carbohydrate (70%), 5.5 grams dietary fiber
22 mg. cholesterol, 351 mg. sodium, $.15

1 raisin-walnut muffin of 10 with 1% fat buttermilk

Exchanges: 0.25 meat, 0.25 milk, 1.25 bread, 0.25 fruit
204 calories, 6.5 grams protein (10%), 5 grams fat (20%)
39 grams carbohydrate (60%), 6 grams dietary fiber
22 mg. cholesterol, 351 mg. sodium, $.25

EMILIE'S DELUXE BRAN MUFFINS

Yum! Good enough for dessert! Top with a dollop of whipped cream for fun!

AMOUNT: 12 large muffins
Bake: 350° for 20 minutes

1. Follow recipe for *Minute Blender Bran Muffins* (p. 356) using:
   1 cup chopped dates or date dices (p. 268)
   1 cup raisins (softened in water, drained)
   1 cup chopped walnuts
   1 cup shredded coconut, unsweetened (optional) (p. 268)

2. To use the blender method, fold all the above into the moistened bran mixture.

3. To use the standard way of mixing (following Variation in Procedure for *Minute Blender Bran Muffins*), fold all the above into the batter after mixing in the bran and the dry ingredients.

4. This recipe makes more batter, so you will need all 12 muffin cups, filled quite full.

1 muffin of 12 with 1% fat buttermilk (no coconut)

Exchanges: 0.5 meat, 1.25 bread, 1 fat, 1.25 fruit
261 calories, 8 grams protein (10%), 17.5 grams fat (23%)
49 grams carbohydrate (61%), 7 grams dietary fiber
19 mg. cholesterol, 294 mg. sodium, $.35

1 muffin of 12 with 1% fat buttermilk (with coconut)

Exchanges: 0.5 meat, 1.25 bread, 1.75 fat, 1.25 fruit
295 calories, 8 grams protein (9%), 10 grams fat (30%)
50 grams carbohydrate (56%), 8.5 grams dietary fiber
19 mg. cholesterol, 296 mg. sodium, $.35

WHOLE-WHEAT POPOVERS

Our children love these and gobble them up, competing over who can get three of them! Great served with soups, they are light and hollow in the centers. Delicious with butter or 100% fruit jam. Do not expect these to rise as high and firm as white flour popovers. Tops of popovers will sink soon after removing from oven, which is normal. Serve immediately after removing from pan. Use the Variation below if you do not have a grain mill or access to fresh whole-grain flour.

AMOUNT: 12 popovers
Bake: 450° for 15 minutes; then 350° for 20 minutes

1. Preheat oven to 450°. Grease muffin pan very well or thoroughly coat with olive oil nonstick spray (if two average-size 12-cup muffin pans available, use the pan with deeper cups).

2. Place in blender and blend on high speed for 30 seconds:

   3 large eggs
   1½ cups low-fat milk
   1 cup whole-wheat pastry flour (p. 267)
   ¾ teaspoon salt (*RealSalt preferred, p. 269*)

3. Pour batter evenly into muffin cups, filling at least ¾ full.

> **Special Tip:** The flour settles quickly to the bottom of the container while pouring. It is thus necessary to stir it up again 2 or 3 times while pouring the batter into the muffin cups. If this seems tedious to do in the blender, pour the batter into a pitcher or quart measure before filling the muffin cups.

4. Bake at 450° for 15 minutes; turn heat down to 350° and continue baking about 20 minutes until golden. Cool 5 minutes before removing from pan. Serve immediately.

VARIATION

In place of whole-wheat pastry flour, use ⅔ **cup whole-wheat pastry grain** (p. 270) in step 2. Blend for 3-4 minutes on high speed. Do not use an aged blender with dull motor or blades. Use a blender that will crush ice cubes. A 10-speed Osterizer works well.

1 popover of 12

Exchanges: 0.25 meat, 0.25 milk, 0.5 bread, 0.5 fat
76 calories, 4 grams protein (19%), 2 grams fat (25%)
11 grams carbohydrate (56%), 1 gram dietary fiber
0 mg. cholesterol, 166 mg. sodium, $.10

PINEAPPLE CORNBREAD
A different version of a familiar recipe!

AMOUNT: 12 servings (8" or 9" square bake pan)
Bake: 350° for 25-30 minutes

1. Preheat oven to 350°. Grease or coat baking pan with olive oil nonstick spray.
2. Whisk together:
   2 eggs or 4 egg whites
   2 tablespoons honey
   20-oz. can unsweetened crushed pineapple, undrained
3. Blend dry ingredients thoroughly in separate bowl:
   3 cups stoneground cornmeal *(p. 267)*
   2 teaspoons baking powder *(low sodium or Rumford, p. 268)*
   1 teaspoon salt *(RealSalt preferred, p. 269)*
4. Blend liquid ingredients into dry ingredients just until mixed. Pour into greased 8" or 9" square pan. Bake 25-35 minutes.

1 piece of 12

Exchanges: 0.25 meat, 1.5 bread, 0.5 fruit
163 calories, 4 grams protein (9%), 2 grams fat (12%)
33 grams carbohydrate (79%), 5 grams dietary fiber
36 mg. cholesterol, 194 mg. sodium, $.25

VARIATIONS
♥ In place of 1 cup cornmeal use:
   1 cup whole-wheat pastry flour *(p. 267)*
♥ Add to either version (all corn, or part wheat):
   2-4 tablespoons melted butter or oil

1 piece of 12—Variation with whole-wheat pastry flour
and 4 tablespoons unsalted butter

Exchanges: 0.25 meat, 1.75 bread, 0.75 fat, 1 fruit
202 calories, 4 grams protein (8%), 6 grams fat (25%)
35 grams carbohydrate (67%), 4.5 grams dietary fiber
46 mg. cholesterol, 195 mg. sodium, $.25

BROCCOLI, ORANGE & FIG SALAD

Be creative in your salads. A bright, colorful salad a little out of the ordinary can transform a meal. The dressing is very light and mild, and is ¹/₄ the volume of the original recipe.

AMOUNT: 4 servings

1. Begin with about **1¹/₂ lbs. broccoli** (untrimmed). Cut flowerets, leaving about 1 inch of the stalk. Cook and drain according to *Cooked Broccoli* (p. 362).

2. Combine and chill thoroughly:

   cooked broccoli flowerets
   2 ribs celery, thinly sliced on diagonal

3. Blend the following ingredients for the dressing, pour over chilled broccoli and celery, and allow to marinate in refrigerator while preparing the remainder of the salad:

   ¹/₂ cup orange juice
   2 tablespoons *Newman's Own Olive Oil & Vinegar Dressing* (p. 268) **or *Emilie's Olive Oil Dressing*** (p. 372) **or Italian dressing**
   1 teaspoon crystalline fructose (p. 268) **or honey**
   ¹/₂ teaspoon dill weed

4. Prepare:

   2 oranges, peeled and cut into half slices
   12 dried black Mission figs, sliced (use scissors)

5. Arrange on individual salad or dinner plates:

   butter lettuce or other leafy lettuce greens
   broccoli and celery mounded in center
   orange slices
   figs mingled among the orange slices
   excess dressing poured over all

1 serving

Exchanges: 1 fat, 3.25 fruit, 1.75 vegetable
287 calories, 7 grams protein (9%), 5.5 grams fat (16%)
60 grams carbohydrate (75%), 7.5 grams dietary fiber
0 mg. cholesterol, 130 mg. sodium, $.90

SNAPPY BEAN SALAD

Colorful and refreshing! My favorite way to cook fresh green beans is in the pressure cooker at 15 lbs. pressure for 2 minutes with ¹/₂ cup water.

AMOUNT: 6 servings

1. Blend together for marinade:

   ¹/₄ cup canola or safflower oil
   2 tablespoons lemon juice *(fresh preferred)*
   1 tablespoon catsup *(no salt added preferred, p. 268)*
   ¹/₂ teaspoon crystalline fructose *(p. 268)* **or honey**
   ¹/₄ teaspoon salt *(RealSalt preferred, p. 269)*
   ¹/₈ teaspoon paprika

2. Combine marinade with remaining ingredients except croutons; refrigerate 1 hour or longer; fold in croutons just before serving:

   2 cups cooked fresh green beans, cut diagonally or 10 oz. frozen cut green beans, cooked
   1 cup cucumber, peeled and cut into small chunks
   2 small tomatoes, wedges cut in half
   8.5-oz. can garbanzo beans *(no salt added preferred)*
   2 green onions, chopped
   1 cup *Soup 'n' Salad Croutons* *(below)*

1 serving of 6 (includes croutons)

Exchanges: 1 bread, 2 fat, 1.25 vegetable
186 calories, 4.5 grams protein (9%), 12 grams fat (53%)
19.5 grams carbohydrate (38%), 4 grams dietary fiber
3 mg. cholesterol, 248 mg. sodium, $.50

SOUP 'N' SALAD CROUTONS

AMOUNT: about 12 cups
Bake: 300° for 20-30 minutes

Toss together and bake in single layer on cookie sheet at 300° until crisp, about 20-30 minutes; stir and rearrange for even toasting if needed. Store in freezer in Ziploc freezer bag:

   1-1¹/₂ lb. loaf whole-grain bread *(p. 267)*
   ¹/₂ cup (1 stick) melted butter *(unsalted preferred)*
   ¹/₈ teaspoon garlic powder
   Spike Seasoning, to taste *(p. 269)*

1 cup:

2.25 bread, 1.5 fat
203 calories, 6 grams protein (11%), 9 grams fat (39%)
27 grams carbohydrate (50%), 6 grams dietary fiber
21 mg. cholesterol, 342 mg. sodium, $.30

COOKED BROCCOLI

A vegetable with more than its share of valuable nutrients. High in vitamins A and C. This cooking method is foolproof for crisp-tender, bright-green broccoli every time. Chill it for use in salads and fresh veggie platters, as well as to serve for a hot vegetable. It keeps well 2 or 3 days in the refrigerator in a tightly covered container.

AMOUNT: 1 lb. per 3 to 4 servings

1. Bring to a boil enough water to cover broccoli.

2. Add cleaned broccoli gradually to the water so that it continues to boil; boil uncovered for 40-60 seconds—no longer! Drain (save the water for soup, if desired).

1-cup serving

Exchanges: 1.75 vegetable
46 calories, 4.5 grams protein (33%), 0.5 gram fat (6%)
9 grams carbohydrate (61%), 3 grams dietary fiber
0 mg. cholesterol, 16 mg. sodium, $.25

STEAMED BROCCOLI

Place broccoli in vegetable steamer basket over boiling water and cook 2 minutes uncovered. Cover and cook until crisp-tender, about 5-10 minutes.

BROCCOLI-CARROT MEDLEY

Add a little interest to plain broccoli by adding julienne-cut carrots.

AMOUNT: 4 servings

1. Wash and trim stalks of outer tough layer, and cut length-wise, leaving about 3" stalk:

   about 1 lb. broccoli

2. Scrub and cut julienne (see below):

   1 medium carrot (about ½ cup)

3. Place carrots in vegetable steamer basket over boiling water, cover and steam 5 minutes; add broccoli, steam uncovered for 2 minutes; cover and steam 5 minutes longer.

4. *Optional:* Blend and pour over vegetables just before serving (this is important as lemon will turn broccoli a sickly yellow-green after a time):

   1 tablespoon melted butter *(unsalted preferred)*
   juice of ½ lemon (or 2 teaspoons)

1 serving of 4 without lemon butter

Exchanges: 1.25 vegetable
31 calories, 3 grams protein (29%), less than 0.5 gram fat (5%)
6 grams carbohydrate (67%), 1.5 grams dietary fiber
0 mg. cholesterol, 30 mg. sodium, $.20

1 serving of 4 with lemon butter

Exchanges: 0.5 fat, 1.25 vegetable
56 calories, 3 grams protein (17%), 3 grams fat (43%)
6.5 grams carbohydrate (40%), 1.5 grams dietary fiber
7 mg. cholesterol, 30 mg. sodium, $.25

JULIENNE-CUT CARROTS

Cutting frequently used vegetables in a variety of ways sparks interest. Cutting carrots julienne takes a little extra time, but gives a gourmet touch. Use a chef's knife.

1. Cut carrot crosswise into fourths.

2. Slice each piece lengthwise into several thin flat strips.

3. Lay each flat strip flat side down on cutting board and cut into thin slivers (some of these may need cutting again).

SUNSHINE SHAKE

A complete low-fat mini-meal in just 5 minutes! A children's cookbook lesson from **Lunches & Snacks**, *this recipe is also demonstrated on our* **"Eating Better with Sue"** *video.*

AMOUNT: 1 or 2 servings (almost 2 cups)

1. Place ingredients in a blender. Follow the special tips given below for cutting and peeling the orange:

   1 medium orange, peeled, chopped
   1 medium banana, peeled, broken into chunks
   ½ cup low-fat plain or vanilla yogurt
   ¹⁄₁₆ teaspoon nutmeg (half of ⅛ teaspoon)
   ¹⁄₁₆ teaspoon cinnamon

2. Cover blender and blend on high speed until mixture is smooth, about 1 minute.

3. To serve, pour into one large or two smaller glasses.

> **Special Tip:** Leave as much of the white pulp on the orange as you can when you peel it. The pulp contains biflavonoids, called vitamin P. Vitamin C works more effectively in the body when eaten with biflavonoids.

Orange Peeling and Cutting Tips

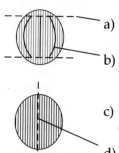

a) Use a cutting board. With a sharp knife slice peeling off each end of orange.

b) Between sliced ends, score around the orange evenly in 5 or 6 places. Use a sharp knife or orange peeler.

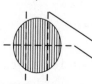

c) With fingers peel away scored sections of peeling from top down.

d) Cut peeled orange in half lengthwise.

e) Cut each half in 3 wedges.

f) Cut wedges in half crosswise.

> **NUTRITION QUIZ:** What 2 nutrient groups does *Sunshine Shake* fit into best? Which ingredients contain fiber? What vitamin is the orange high in? Name one valuable mineral found in bananas. (Answers are on p. 366.) What kind of sugar makes this recipe taste sweet? Is it low-fat? (Answers are on p. 381.)

ORANGE FROSTY

A winner with children. Perfect after-school refresher on a hot afternoon! A lesson from the Children's Cookbook section of **Lunches & Snacks**. *Be sure the blender you use is the type that will crush ice cubes.*

AMOUNT: about 4 cups

1. Place ingredients in a blender in the following order:

   6-oz. can frozen orange juice concentrate, unsweetened
   6-oz. juice can (³/₄ cup) low-fat milk
   ¹/₄ cup noninstant nonfat dry milk powder *(p. 269)*
   1 banana, peeled, broken
   ¹/₄ teaspoon vanilla extract
   ice cubes to fill up blender

2. Cover blender and blend on high speed until ice cubes are completely crushed, about 30 seconds.

3. To serve, fill glasses and drink immediately. This drink does not store well in the refrigerator. Drink slowly! You might want to "eat" it with a spoon.

> **Special Tip:** Leftover *Orange Frosty* makes yummy popsicles!

> **NUTRITION QUIZ:** What 2 nutrient groups does *Orange Frosty* fit into best? Can you think of 3 reasons why this drink is healthier than soda pop? Look at the chart below. How do *Orange Frosty* and *Sunshine Shake* (prepared with vanilla yogurt) compare in amount of calories, protein, carbohydrates, fiber, and cost? Are these low-fat recipes? Do they cost more than a can of soda pop? (Answers are on p. 381.)

1-cup serving	Sunshine Shake	Orange Frosty
calories	150 calories	160 calories
protein	4.7 grams	5.8 grams
carbohydrate	32.6 grams	33 grams
fat	1.2 grams	1.1 grams
fat % of calories	7%	6%
dietary fiber	2.3 grams	0.9 grams
cholesterol	4 milligrams	5 milligrams
sodium	43 milligrams	65 milligrams
cost	$.27	$.28

FRUIT SMOOTHIE

A dairyless, delicious, filling shake from **Breakfasts!** *Cut recipe in half for 1 sumptuous serving.*

AMOUNT: 2 to 4 servings

Place in blender and blend until smooth:

2 frozen or unfrozen bananas, broken in chunks
1 cup *Alice's Fruit Soup* (p. 367)
1 orange, peeled, cut in chunks
3-4 ice cubes

1 serving of 2:

Exchanges: 3.5 fruit
209 calories, 2.5 grams protein (5%), 1 gram fat (4%)
52 grams carbohydrate (91%), 6.5 grams dietary fiber
0 mg. cholesterol, 7 mg. sodium, $.70

VARIATIONS

♥ For sweeter shake add ¼ **cup frozen juice concentrate** (any flavor desired).

♥ In place of *Alice's Fruit Soup*, add:
an extra orange
1 apple
6 chopped dates or a handful of date dices (p. 268)
¼ cup frozen fruit-juice concentrate, unsweetened (such as banana-pineapple, or banana-orange-pineapple)
water to the 1-cup mark (after all the other ingredients are added to the blender)

1 serving of 2 (Variation with frozen fruit-juice concentrate, dates, extra orange, apple):

Exchanges: 5.75 fruit
352 calories, 3.5 grams protein (3%), 1 gram fat (3%)
88 grams carbohydrate (94%), 8 grams dietary fiber
0 mg. cholesterol, 8 mg. sodium, $.70

ALICE'S FRUIT SOUP

A so-o-o refreshing 5-minute recipe from **Breakfasts!** *Delicious as a waffle topping, a fruit snack, or a dessert topped with whipped cream. Use the leftovers for Fruit Smoothie, p. 366. Vary any of the fruits except the raspberries, but substitute frozen for frozen, and canned for canned.*

AMOUNT: 11 cups (without bananas)

1. Place in a large bowl:

   12-oz. package frozen raspberries
   16-oz. package frozen strawberries
   12-oz. package frozen blueberries, boysenberries, or black-berries

2. Add and stir to combine:

   20-oz. can pineapple chunks, unsweetened, undrained
   16-oz. can peach slices, unsweetened, undrained (cut up)
   16-oz. can pear halves, unsweetened, undrained (cut up)

3. Let stand about 2 hours at room temperature or overnight in refrigerator to let frozen fruit thaw and juices mingle.

4. Refrigerate until ready to serve. Add to portion to be served:

   sliced bananas, as desired (optional)

1-cup serving (banana not included)

Exchanges: 2 fruit
118 calories, 1 gram protein (4%), 0.5 gram fat (4%)
30 grams carbohydrate (93%), 4.5 grams dietary fiber
0 mg. cholesterol, 8 mg. sodium, $.80

1-cup serving plus ¼ cup banana slices

Exchanges 2.5 fruit
155 calories, 1.5 grams protein (4%), 0.5 gram fat (4%)
39 grams carbohydrate (92%), 5.5. grams dietary fiber
0 mg. cholesterol, 13 mg. sodium, $.85

EMILIE'S YUMMY OATMEALS

Rich and delicious morsels from Desserts that stand up in little mounds. These contain "the works!"

AMOUNT: about 4 dozen (5 dozen with coconut)
Bake: 350° for 10-12 minutes

1. Preheat oven to 350°. Grease or spray cookie sheet.

2. Whisk butter and honey together until well blended and creamy; whisk in egg:

   1 stick (¹/₂ cup) soft butter *(unsalted preferred)*
   ²/₃ cup honey
   1 egg

3. Blend dry ingredients in a separate bowl:

   1 cup whole-wheat pastry flour *(p. 267)*
   1 teaspoon cinnamon
   ¹/₂ teaspoon baking soda
   ¹/₂ teaspoon salt *(RealSalt preferred, p. 269)*
   ¹/₄ teaspoon nutmeg

4. With mixing spoon stir dry ingredients into liquid ingredients just until evenly mixed.

5. Mix in evenly:

   2 cups *Quick Quaker Oats*, uncooked
   1 cup raisins
   1 cup carob chips *(p. 268)* **or chocolate chips**
   1 cup date dices *(p. 268)* **or chopped dates**
   1 cup chopped walnuts
   1 cup coconut, unsweetened (optional)—**medium or fine shredded** *(p. 268)*

6. Drop by tablespoonfuls onto lightly greased cookie sheet, spacing close together. If dough does not hold together well, press each dropped cookie together a bit with fingertips.

7. Bake at 350° for 10-12 minutes. Cool before removing from cookie sheet.

---

1 cookie without coconut (amounts almost the same with coconut added)

Exchanges: 0.5 bread, 0.75 fat, 0.5 fruit (0.25 fruit with coconut)
109 calories (94 with coconut), 2.5 grams protein (8%), 5 grams fat (36%)
16 grams carbohydrate (56%), 1.5 grams dietary fiber
10 mg. cholesterol, 33 mg. sodium, $.15

ORANGE OR LEMON SPICE COOKIES

A delicate spice flavor with a hint of orange or lemon. These cookies will be crisp with Sucanat (granulated evaporated whole sugar cane juice—see p. 269), soft with honey. Sue's favorite cookie! Wheatless alternatives for wheat flour in cookies is available from **Desserts** *(see p. 384).*

AMOUNT: about 2¹/₂ dozen
Bake: 375° for 8-10 minutes

1. Preheat oven to 375°. Grease or spray cookie sheet.
2. Whisk together until thoroughly blended:
   1 stick (¹/₂ cup) very soft butter (unsalted preferred)
   1 cup Sucanat (health-food store) **or ¹/₂ cup honey**
3. Whisk in until well blended:
   1 egg
   1 teaspoon vanilla
4. Blend dry ingredients in separate bowl; stir into liquid ingredients (dough will be quite stiff with Sucanat):
   2 cups whole-wheat pastry flour (p. 267)
   1 tablespoon noninstant nonfat dry milk powder (p. 269)
   1 tablespoon grated lemon or orange peel
   ¹/₂ teaspoon cinnamon
   ¹/₂ teaspoon nutmeg
   1 teaspoon baking powder (low sodium or Rumford, p. 268)
   ¹/₂ teaspoon baking soda
5. Chill dough for easy handling. Drop by tablespoonfuls onto greased cookie sheet, leaving room for spreading (these usually spread quite a bit).
6. Flatten shaped dough slightly on cookie sheet with floured fork.
7. Sprinkle each cookie with **cinnamon sugar** (optional—see below) and top with an **almond**.
8. Bake in preheated oven at 375° for 8-10 minutes until lightly browned. Cool 2 minutes before removing from cookie sheet.

1 cookie of 2¹/₂ dozen with ¹/₈ teaspoon cinnamon sugar and 1 almond

Exchanges: 0.5 bread, 0.75 fat
92 calories, 1.5 grams protein (6%), 4 grams fat (38%)
13.5 grams carbohydrate (56%), 1 gram dietary fiber
15 mg. cholesterol, 18 mg. sodium, $.15

Cinnamon Sugar: Blend **5 tablespoons crystalline fructose** with **2 teaspoons cinnamon**. Store in a spice shaker bottle.

FROZEN VANILLA YOGURT

A crunchy ice frost from Desserts.

AMOUNT: 2 cups

1. Liquefy in blender:

    2 cups nonfat or low-fat plain yogurt
    ¼ cup crystalline fructose *(p. 268)*
    1 teaspoon vanilla

2. Pour into bowl or tray; freeze until set.

3. Scoop into electric mixer; beat until soft.

4. Refreeze until set.

5. Allow to stand at room temperature about 10 minutes before serving.

½ cup with nonfat yogurt

Exchanges: 0.5 milk; 98 calories, 6.5 grams protein (25%)
19 grams carbohydrate (73%), 2 mg. cholesterol, 67 mg. sodium, $.35

PINEAPPLE TOPPING

Plain crushed pineapple makes a tasty topping for frozen yogurt, ice cream, or waffles. If you want a little thicker and sweeter topping, try this simple recipe.

AMOUNT: 2½ cups

1. Blend together in saucepan with wire whisk:

    20-oz. can crushed pineapple, unsweetened
    1½ tablespoons arrowroot powder *(p. 268)* **or cornstarch**
    1 tablespoon honey or crystalline fructose, to taste *(p. 268)*

2. Bring to a very low boil over medium heat, stirring constantly. Cook and stir about 1 minute until thickened (watch carefully—pineapple burns easily).

¼ cup

Exchanges: 0.5 fruit
46 calories, 11 grams carbohydrate (98%), 0.5 grams dietary fiber
0 mg. cholesterol, 1 mg. sodium, $.10

VARIATION

For a smaller recipe (1 cup) use **8-oz. can crushed pineapple, 2 teaspoons arrowroot powder or cornstarch, 1½ teaspoons honey or crystalline fructose.**

PATTY'S CURRY DIP

*From the kitchen of my sister, Patty, an excellent cook. Chilling improves flavor. Also tasty as a salad dressing. From **Lunches & Snacks**.*

AMOUNT: about 1½ cups

1. Blend all together with wire whisk:

   ¾ **cup nonfat or low-fat yogurt**
   ¾ **cup light sour cream or sour cream**
   1½ **teaspoons curry powder**
   1 teaspoon dill weed
   ½ **teaspoon soy sauce** *(Kikkoman Lite preferred, p. 269)*
   ¼ **teaspoon tarragon** *(optional)*
   ⅛ **teaspoon onion powder or 1 tablespoon minced onion**
   1/16 **teaspoon salt** *(RealSalt preferred, p. 269)*
   1 to 2 teaspoons lemon juice, to taste

2. Chill before serving.

1 tablespoon
Exchanges: 0.25 fat
16 calories, 1 gram protein (22%), 1 gram fat (48%)
1 gram carbohydrate (29%)
3 mg. cholesterol, 20 mg. sodium, $.05

BUTTER SPREAD

*Combine saturated and unsaturated fat for a balanced fat spread! Avoids the hydrogenated fat of margarines. Canola oil provides a good balance of both essential fatty acids—linoleic and linolenic plus a high portion of monounsaturated fat. Stays spreadable directly from the refrigerator, but don't leave it out too long or it will return to a semi-liquid state. Make whatever amount you desire using equal portions of butter and oil. Add a little salt, to taste. Recipe from **Breakfasts**.*

AMOUNT: 1 cup

1. Whisk together, gradually adding oil to butter until smooth and no lumps:

   1 stick (½ cup) lightly salted butter, very soft
   ½ **cup canola oil**
   1 tablespoon liquid lecithin (optional) *(health-food store)*

2. Refrigerate in covered container.

1-tablespoon (lecithin not included)
Exchanges: 2.5 fat; 110 calories, 13 grams fat (100%)
16 mg. cholesterol, 58 mg. sodium, $.10

EMILIE'S OLIVE OIL DRESSING

Emilie's best dressing recipe from her Viennese-chef father. Always a winner!

AMOUNT: 1½ cups

1. Mash together with tip of a knife and put in pint jar:

   3 cloves garlic, pressed
   1 teaspoon salt *(RealSalt preferred, p. 269)*
   ½ scant teaspoon pepper

2. Add and shake well; chill:

   1 cup olive oil
   ½ cup wine vinegar
   juice of 1 lemon (about ¼ cup)

1-tablespoon serving
Exchanges: 1.5 fat
70 calories, 8 grams fat (98%), 76 mg. sodium, $.10

THOUSAND ISLAND DRESSING

Use yogurt to stretch mayonnaise for a lower-fat dressing or spread.

AMOUNT: 2½ cups

Blend together with a wire whisk:

   1¼ cups nonfat plain yogurt
   ¾ cup mayonnaise *(p. 269)*
   ¼ cup catsup *(no salt added preferred, p. 268)*
   1 tablespoon lemon juice
   1½ teaspoons crystalline fructose *(p. 268)*
   ¼ teaspoon salt (optional)
   ⅛ teaspoon garlic powder
   1 small dill pickle, chopped fine or
       1-2 tablespoons sweet pickle relish

1-tablespoon serving
Exchanges: 0.75 fat
38 calories, 0.5 gram protein (4%), 3.5 grams fat (87%)
1 gram carbohydrate (8%), 2 mg. cholesterol, 42 mg. sodium, $.05

SUE'S HOUSE DRESSING

A creamy reduced-fat dressing!

AMOUNT: 1¹/₂ cups

Blend thoroughly with wire whisk:

> **1 cup nonfat or low-fat plain yogurt**
> **¹/₂ cup mayonnaise** *(p. 269)*
> **1 tablespoon lemon juice**
> **¹/₂ teaspoon fresh or dried parsley or chives**
> **¹/₂ teaspoon onion powder**
> **¹/₄ teaspoon salt** (optional) *(RealSalt preferred, p. 269)*
> **¹/₈ teaspoon garlic powder**

1-tablespoon serving
Exchanges: 0.75 fat
41 calories, 0.5 gram protein (5%), 4 grams fat (89%)
0.5 gram carbohydrate (6%)
0 mg. cholesterol, 55 mg. sodium, $.05

SWEET LITE DRESSING

A simple and refreshing fat-free, low-calorie dressing for coleslaws and tossed salads with fruit. One-fourth cup is about right for a salad for 4 persons.

AMOUNT: ¹/₄ cup

Blend thoroughly with wire whisk:

> **¹/₄ cup nonfat yogurt**
> **2 teaspoons crystalline fructose** *(p. 268)* **or honey**
> **2 teaspoons lemon juice**
> **¹/₈ teaspoon salt** *(RealSalt preferred, p. 269)*

1-tablespoon serving
Exchanges: negligible
14 calories, 3 grams carbohydrate (76%), 75 mg. sodium, $.05

SWEET ORANGE DRESSING

Surprisingly refreshing, tasty, effortless, and so-o-o nonfat! Good on most salads, including tossed salads.

Squeeze and pour over salad, tossing lightly:

> **juice of ¹/₂ orange**
> **(That's right! Just the juice of half an orange!)**

juice of ¹/₂ orange
Exchanges: 0.5 fruit
31 calories, 7.5 grams carbohydrate (90%), $.10

PINEAPPLE SUNSHINE MOLD

The base of unsweetened orange juice and pineapple juice sweetened with honey makes a good gelatin salad. Tasty with yogurt blended with sour cream.

AMOUNT: 8 to 10 servings (8-9" square or 9" x 13" pan)

1. In small saucepan, whisk gelatin into juice to soften and let stand 5 minutes:

   ³/₄ cup orange juice
   1 envelope (2 teaspoons) unflavored gelatine

2. Meanwhile, mix together in mixing bowl:

   8-oz. can unsweetened crushed pineapple, undrained
   6-oz. can unsweetened pineapple juice
   1 orange, peeled and chopped
   1 banana, peeled and sliced
   ³/₄ cup chopped pecans or almonds (optional)

3. Heat gelatin mixture over medium heat, stirring constantly until dissolved. Remove from heat and blend in:

   3 tablespoons honey

4. Whisk gelatin mixture into remaining ingredients. Pour into 8" or 9" square pan or 9" x 13" pan; chill until set.

5. Cut into squares for individual servings and garnish as desired with **mint leaves, whole strawberries, yogurt-sour cream topping** (half plain yogurt and half sour cream).

1 serving of 8 with pecans (garnish not included)

Exchanges: 0.5 fat, 1 fruit
92 calories, 2 grams protein (7%), 3 grams fat (27%)
16 grams carbohydrate (66%), 1 gram dietary fiber
0 mg. cholesterol, 3 mg. sodium, $.30

1 serving of 8 without nuts (garnish not included)

Exchanges: 1 fruit
66 calories, 1.5 grams protein (8%), less than 0.5 gram fat (3%)
16 grams carbohydrate (89%), 1 gram dietary fiber
0 mg. cholesterol, 3 mg. sodium, $.20

VARIATIONS

♥ Add ¹/₂ **cup Thompson seedless grapes**, cut in half.
♥ Omit banana and orange; add ³/₄ **cup celery** and ³/₄ **cup grated carrot**.

Notes

Chapter 6—Whatever Happened to the Basic Four?
1. *Understanding Vitamins and Minerals: The Prevention Total Health System*, editors of *Prevention Magazine* (Emmaus, PA: Rodale Press, 1984), p. 6.

Chapter 7—God's Cornucopia of Whole Foods
1. Percentage losses adapted from: Ethel Renwick, *Let's Try Real Food* (Grand Rapids, MI: Zondervan Publishing House, 1976), p. 29, and Audrey Eyton, *The F-Plan Diet* (New York: Crown Publishers, 1973), pp. 79-80.

Chapter 13—Overcoming the Four Fears: What About Cost?
1. Bonnie Liebman, "Burgerland Revisited," *Nutrition Action Healthletter*, 12:5 (Washington, DC: Center for Science in the Public Interest, June 1985), p. 1.

Chapter 19—Making Friends with Fiber
1. "Is Fat More Fattening?" *Diet & Nutrition Letter*, 4:12 (New York: Tufts University, Feb. 1987), p. 2.

Chapter 21—The Slippery Subject of Fats
1. Warren N. Levin, "What's the Story on Fats?" *Your Health* (Overland Park, KS: International Academy of Preventive Medicine, Jan. 1984), p. 1.
2. "More Superfoods," *Nutrition News*, 4:12 (Pomona, CA, 1981), p. 1.
3. Kerry Pechter, "The Amazing Benefits of the New Fiber Supplements," *Prevention Magazine* (Emmaus, PA: Rodale Press, Oct. 1982), p. 27.

Chapter 22—Is Meat a Menace to Your Health?
1. "4 to 10 Chickens on Market Contaminated, Says USDA," *Press-Enterprise* (Riverside County, CA, Feb. 19, 1987), p. A-1.
2. "U.S.A. 1971–1983 Estimated Association with Salmonella Illnesses," distributed by Raymond A. Novell, attorney for Alta-Dena Dairy (1085 West Badillo, Covina, CA 91722).
3. Elaine Blume, "Germ Wars," *Nutrition Action Healthletter*, 13:6 (Washington, DC: Center for Science in the Public Interest, June 1986), p. 4.
4. John A. Scharffenberg, *Problems with Meat* (Santa Barbara, CA: Woodbridge Press Publishing Company, 1979), p. 33.
5. Gary Null, *The New Vegetarian* (New York: William Morrow and Company, 1978), p. 19.

6. Weston Price, D.D.S. *Nutrition and Physical Degeneration* (La Mesa, CA: The Price-Pottenger Nutrition Foundation, 1979), p. 279.

Chapter 23—Eggs—Ample of Controversy!
1. Gladys Lindberg and Judy Lindberg McFarland, *Take Charge of Your Health* (San Francisco: Harper & Row Publishers, 1982), pp. 79-80.
2. "Hold the Eggs and Butter," *Time* (Mar. 26, 1984), p. 58.
3. Ibid.
4. Null, *The New Vegetarian*, p. 121.
5. Lindberg and McFarland, *Take Charge of Your Health*, p. 80.

Chapter 24—Are Dairy Products Deadly?
1. Null, *The New Vegetarian*, p. 89.
2. Bernard Jensen, "Raw Milk vs. Pasteurized Milk," *Health Freedom News* (National Health Federation, May 1985), p. 41 and "Which Do You Choose?" Alta-Dena Dairy printed brochure.
3. Frances M. Pottenger, Jr., "The Effect of Heat-Processed Foods and Metabolized Vitamin D Milk on the Dentofacial Structures of Experimental Animals" (Reprinted from *American Journal of Orthodontics and Oral Surgery*, St. Louis, Vol. 32, No. 8, Oral Surgery pages 467-85, Aug. 1946), p. 9.
4. Jensen, *Health Freedom News*, p. 41.
5. "U.S.A. 1971–1983 Estimated Association with Salmonella Illnesses," distributed by Raymond A. Novell, attorney for Alta-Dena Dairy (1085 West Badillo, Covina, CA 91722).
6. "Hold the Eggs and Butter," p. 62.
7. S.I. McMillen, *None of These Diseases* (Charlotte, NC: Commission Press, 1979), pp. 14-16.
8. Weston A. Price, *Nutrition and Physical Degeneration* (La Mesa, CA: The Price-Pottenger Nutrition Foundation, 1970), p. 291.

Chapter 26—The Sensation of Sugar
1. "Sugar and Breast Cancer," *Better Nutrition* (Atlanta: Communications Channels, Inc., July 1983), pp. 13-14ff.
2. Frances Sheridan Goulart, "Sugar Substitutes," *The Herbalist* (Nov. 1979), p. 21.

Chapter 28—A Salty Sermon
1. Ruth Adams, "Does Excessive Salt Cause High Blood Pressure?" *Better Nutrition* (Atlanta: Communications Channels, Inc., May 1985), p. 23.
2. Ibid.
3. Ibid., p. 37.

Chapter 29—I'm Sick and Tired of Being Fat!
1. Bonnie F. Liebman, "Fated to Be Fat?" *Nutrition Action Healthletter* (Washington, DC: Center for Science in the Public Interest, Jan./Feb. 1987), p. 1.

Chapter 30—Exercise: Nutrition's Twin
1. Martin Katahn, Ph.D. *Beyond Diet* (New York: Berkley Books, 1984), pp. 51-53.

Chapter 31—Drink Your Way to Health
1. Firsby, ND, D.Sc., Bill, *God's HMO (Health Maintenance Organization)* (Farmington Hills, MI: Health Support Ministries, 1990), p. 91.

Chapter 32—Mind, Mood, and Food
1. Bernard Fensterwald, III, NNF Legislative Counsel, "Washington Watch—Fighting Crime with Nutrition," *Health Food Review* (Apr. 1983), p. 72.

Chapter 36—Questions Often Asked
1. Ruth Bircher, *Eating Your Way to Health* (London: Faber and Faber, 1961), pp. 32-33.
2. Letitia Brewster and Michael Jacobson, *The Changing American Diet* (Washington, DC: Center for Science in the Public Interest, 1983), p. 1.
3. Elaine Blume and Michael F. Jacobson, "Food Irradiation: Is the Time Ripe?" *Nutrition Action Healthletter* (Washington, DC: Center for Science in the Public Interest, Nov. 1986), p. 7.

Chapter 37—The Value of the Human Body
1. John White, *Masks of Melancholy* (Downers Grove, IL: InterVarsity Press, 1982), p. 41.
2. Ibid., p. 42.

Chapter 38—God Has a Plan for Health
1. *The Relation of Christian Faith to Health*, adopted by the 172nd General Assembly, May 1960 (The United Presbyterian Church in the United States of America, Board of National Missions, 475 Riverside Drive, New York, NY 10027), p. 39.
2. Ibid., p. 38.

Chapter 39—Prevention, Miracle, and Medicine
1. *The Relation of Christian Faith to Health*, adopted by the 172nd General Assembly, May 1960 (The United Presbyterian Church in the

United States of America, Board of National Missions, 475 Riverside Drive, New York, NY 10027), p. 39.
2. Ibid., p. 56.

Chapter 40—Not for Health's Sake
1. Dr. Hans Diehl, *To Your Health* (Redlands, CA: The Quiet Hour, 1987), p. 190.
2. Lindberg, *Take Charge of Your Health*, p. 14.

Chapter 41—The Perfect Vegetarian Diet in the New Age
1. *The Higher Taste* (based on the teachings of A.C. Bhaktivedanta Swami Prabhupada, founder of the International Society for Krishna Consciousness (Los Angeles: The Bhaktivedanta Book Trust, 1984), p. 52.
2. Ibid., p. 51.
3. Ibid.
4. Ibid., p. 52.
5. Ibid., p. 53.
6. Ibid., p. 52.
7. Ibid.
8. Ibid.
9. Ibid., p. 53.

Chapter 42—The Great New Age Health Deception
1. Carol McGraw, "Seekers of Self Now Herald the 'New Age,'" *Los Angeles Times* (Feb. 17, 1987), p. I-17.
2. Ibid., p. 16.
3. Ibid.
4. Laurel Robertson, Carol Flinders, and Bronwen Godfrey, *Laurel's Kitchen* (Berkeley, CA: Nilgiri Press, 1976), p. 46.

Chapter 46—Good Food Is Good for Love
1. Frances Moore Lappe, *Diet for a Small Planet*, Tenth Anniversary Edition (New York: Ballantine Books, 1982), p. 152.
2. Daniel Doriani, "Wasn't The Lord's Supper Originally a Feast?" *Christianity Today*, Mar. 18, 1983, p. 44.

Chapter 47—Christian Ministry in a Hungry World
1. D.B. Jelliffe, "Commerciogenic Malnutrition?" *Nutritional Reviews*, 30:9 (Sep. 1972), p. 43.

Chapter 49—Planning Is a Privilege
1. Keith Green, lyrics from "So You Wanna Go Back to Egypt?" (Sparrow Records, Inc.).

Recommended Reading

Additives

Winter, Ruth. *A Consumer's Dictionary of Food Additives*. New York: Crown Publishers, Inc., new third revised edition, 1989.

Allergies

Henderson, Ph.D., Louise and Ludeman, Ph.D., Kate. *Do-It-Yourself Allergy Analysis Handbook*. New Canaan, CT: Keats Publishing, Inc., 1992.

Biblical Health Standards

Frisby, ND, D.Sc., Bill. *God's HMO (Health Maintenance Organization)*, 23769 Barfield, Farmington Hills, MI 48336: Health-Support Ministries, 1990 (mail order: send $5.00 + $2.00 shipping and handling).

McMillen, S.I. *None of These Diseases*. Old Tappan, NJ: Fleming H. Revell Company, 1983.

Omartian, Stormie. *Greater Health God's Way: Seven Steps to Health, Youthfulness and Vitality*. Canoga Park, CA: Sparrow Press, 1984.

Children & Infants, Feeding & Teaching

Gregg, Sue. *Eating Better with Sue Video Cooking Course*. Riverside, CA: Eating Better Cookbooks, 1987 (see p. 383 for mail order).

Gregg, Sue. *Eating Better Lunches & Snacks: with Lessons for Children*. Riverside, CA: Eating Better Cookbooks, 1991 (see p. 384 for mail order).

La Leche League International. *The Womanly Art of Breastfeeding*, 35th Anniversary Edition. P.O. Box 1209, Franklin Park, IL 60131-8209 USA: La Leche League International, 1991.

McEntire, Patricia. *Mommy, I'm Hungry*. P.O. Box 22246, Sacramento, CA 95822: Cougar Books, 1982.

Exercise & Weight Management

Katahn, Martin. *Beyond Diet*. New York: Berkley Books, 1984.

Fasting

Omartian, Stormie. *Greater Health God's Way: Seven Steps to Health, Youthfulness and Vitality*. Canoga Park, CA: Sparrow Press, 1984.

Wallis, Arthur. *God's Chosen Fast*. Ft. Washington, PA: Christian Literature Crusade, 1974.

Foods, About

Carper, Jean. *The Food Pharmacy*. New York: Bantam Books, 1988.

Finnegan, John. *The Facts About Fats: A Consumer's Guide to Good Oils*. Berkeley, CA: Celestial Arts, 1993.

Wood, Rebecca. *The Whole Foods Encyclopedia*. New York: Prentice Hall Press, 1988.

Food Safety

Jacobson, Ph.D., Michael and Lefferts, Lisa Y. and Garland, Anne Witte: Center for Science in the Public Interest. *Safe Food: Eating Wisely in a Risky World*. Los Angeles: Living Planet Press, 1991.

Webb, Tony and Lang, Tim and Tucker, Kathleen. *Food Irradiation: Who Wants It?* Rochester, VT: Thorsons Publishers, Inc., 1987.

Foods for Healing

Balch, C.N.C., Phyllis A. and Balch, M.D., James F. *Rx Prescription for Cooking & Dietary Wellness: The Wellness Book of the 1990's*. 610 West Main Street, Greenfield, IN 46140: P.A.B. Publishing, Inc., 1987 (revised 1992).

Balch, M.D., James F. and Balch, C.N.C., Phyllis A. *Prescription for Nutritional Healing: A Practical A-Z Reference*. Garden City Park, NY: Avery Publishing Group, Inc., 1990.

Hauseman, Patricia and Benn Hurley, Judith. *The Healing Foods*. Emmaus, PA: Rodale Press, 1989.

Food Storage

Bailey, Janet. *Keeping Food Fresh*. Garden City, NY: The Dial Press, 1985.

Jewish Feasts for Christian Instruction & Celebration

Gregg, Sue. *Holiday Menus*. Riverside, CA: Eating Better Cookbooks, 1989 (includes healthy Passover seder menu; see p. 383 for mail order).

Kinard, Malvina and Crisler, Janet. *Loaves & Fishes: Foods from Bible Times*. New Canaan, CT: Keats Publishing, Inc., 1975.

Zimmerman, Martha. *Celebrate the Feasts*. Minneapolis, MN: Bethany House Publishers, 1975.

Juicing

Kordich, Jay. *The Juiceman's Power of Juicing*. New York: William Morrow and Company, Inc., 1992.

New Age Vegetarianism

Maharaj, Rabi R. *Death of a Guru*. Eugene, OR: Harvest House Publishers, 1984.

Shopping

Goldbeck, Nikki and Goldbeck, David. *The Supermarket Handbook*. New York: New American Library, 1976.

Vitamins/Minerals

Nutrition Search, Inc. *Nutrition Almanac*. New York: McGraw-Hill Book Co., 1979.

World Effects of the Western Diet

Price, D.D.S., Weston A. *Nutrition and Physical Degeneration*. LaMesa, CA: The Price-Pottenger Nutrition Foundation, 1970 (mail order only; order brochure: P.O. Box 2614, La Mesa, CA 92044-2614). Invaluable book, especially for missionaries!

NUTRITION QUIZ ANSWERS

Sunshine Shake	*Orange Frosty*
1. Carbohydrates and proteins	1. Carbohydrates and proteins
2. Vitamin C	2. Has fiber, protein, and vitamin C
3. Potassium	3. See chart on page 365 for answer
4. Fructose	4. Yes
5. Yes	5. No

Recipe Index

More Cooking and Home Ideas from Sue and Emilie

Additional cooking helps and materials available from Sue Gregg's *Eating Better Cookbooks:*

- ♥ *Eating Better Cooking Course*
- ♥ *The "Eating Better with Sue" video*
- ♥ *Holiday Menus* book
- ♥ *The Creative Recipe Organizer*
- ♥ *Sue's "Kitchen Magic" Seasoning*
- ♥ *Yeast Breads* book (for use with bread-kneader machines)
- ♥ *Quantity Recipes* book (for cooking with large groups)
- ♥ *Taste & Tell Dining* menu plans and handout recipes

For a current price list, please send your name and address along with two first-class stamps to:

Sue Gregg's Eating Better Cookbooks
8830 Glencoe Drive
Riverside, CA 92503
1-909-687-5491

Other helpful books on home organization and creativity by Emilie Barnes, founder of the popular "More Hours in My Day" seminars:

- ♥ *The 15-Minute Organizer*
- ♥ *The 15-Minute Money Manager*
- ♥ *15 Minutes Alone with God*
- ♥ *Survival for Busy Women*
- ♥ *The Creative Home Organizer*
- ♥ *The Complete Holiday Organizer*
- ♥ *My Prayer Planner*
- ♥ *More Hours in My Day*
- ♥ *The Spirit of Loveliness*
- ♥ *If Teacups Could Talk*

For additional information and a current price list, send your request and a stamped, self-addressed envelope to:

More Hours in My Day
2838 Rumsey Drive
Riverside, CA 92506

Sue Gregg's
Eating Better Cookbooks

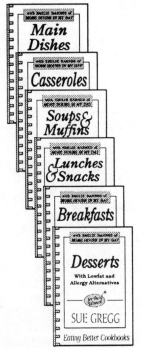

Main Dishes *with over 100 Complete Menus* includes over 270 recipes and 138 menus, with 52 low-budget meals and 58 low-fat meals that average just 20% fat (of calories). Vegetarian alternatives. 292 pgs.

Casseroles Meals in Minutes is a whole-foods convenience cookbook that stocks your freezer. Five sets of 5 recipes with menus, shopping, and assembly lists. Chicken, fish, turkey, bean, and vegetarian recipes. 90 pgs.

Soups & Muffins provides 36 muffin recipes from 12 whole grains. Alternatives for wheat and dairy allergies; 27 soup recipes nutritionally improved. 102 pgs.

Breakfasts *with Blender Batter Baking and Allergy Alternatives* introduces incredibly easy whole-grain blender batters for light waffles and pancakes, coffee cakes, muffins, and crepes. 312 pgs.

Lunches & Snacks *with Lessons for Children* includes a young cook's guide on food preparation with nutritional helps. 168 pgs.

Desserts *with Low-Fat and Allergy Alternatives* supplies recipes to satisfy the sweet tooth without white flour, white sugar, or hydrogenated fats. Forty-five recipes under 200 calories and 30% fat. 175 pgs.

Complete Index & Menu Planner references all six volumes so you can find recipes quickly. Recipes categorized by type for monthly menu planning.